THIS BOOK about allergy plants is written for the suffering people (10 to 20 percent of the population) who are tormented by these interesting but often inconspicuous plants. Plants causing allergies are difficult to identify because they seldom have prominent flowers. These plants sometimes appear in weed identification guides but usually not in wildflower books. Some are only found in rare monographs.

You cannot hide from allergy plants by staying in the big cities. Allergenic plants grow abundantly in areas where man is disturbing the natural environment for his homes, roadways, and agricultural activities. Very few of the highly allergenic plants are found in virgin forests, mountains, or swamps. They grow best in soil disturbed by man's activities.

It is almost impossible to avoid plants which cause allergies, because pollen can travel many miles on the breezes. However, the ability to avoid large doses is critical for sensitive people. The intensity of the allergic reaction depends on the amount of exposure.

This book is designed to help allergy sufferers recognize the cause of their misery, the allergenic plants. Jaw-breaking botanical words have been avoided when possible. However, scientific names must be used to be certain of the identity of plants. It would be more comfortable to use common names, but there are so many different common names for most plants that the use of these names might cause confusion.

What is an allergy?

The exact nature of allergy is a mystery to many people. Allergy is an abnormal reaction to a very small amount of a specific substance, called an allergen.* This substance is harmless to people who do not have this particular allergy. Allergens stimulate the production of allergic antibodies or of sensitized cells.

Allergens may be contained in pollens, molds, animal skin cells, house dust, insects, medications, or even foods such as fish, eggs, milk, citrus, berries, wheat or nuts. These allergens cause trouble when they are inhaled (pollens, dust, and spores), swallowed (food), or injected into the body (some drugs and insect venoms). This book is primarily concerned with the most common cause of allergy, airborne plant pollen.

One reaction upon exposure to these pollen allergens is "hay fever,"** a condition in which the lining of the nose becomes swollen and exudes a watery discharge, the nose and palate itch, and there are frequent sneezes. The eyes may become itchy, reddened, and runny, and some persons may proceed to chronic ear infections.

Another reaction to allergens is "asthma." In "asthma" there may be difficulty in breathing, with a wheezing sound as the air passes through narrowed airways.

There are other allergic reactions such as hives, severe edema (swelling caused by fluid collecting in the tissues), and shock. These seldom occur from ordinary exposure to allergy plants.

A person without allergies exposed to these allergens has no reaction.

Allergens are so small that they are not usually seen, and thus it often seems mysterious that the allergic person can detect such a small amount of the allergen. Just a brief contact with some plants can result in rashes, as with poison ivy, which stimulates a delayed allergic reaction. The itching, weeping rash appears 24-48 hours after the poison ivy plant has been touched.

---

*Allergens are usually proteins or glycoproteins of a molecular weight of 10,000 to 60,000.

**The expression "hay fever" is a misnomer. "Hay fever" is neither caused by hay, nor is there any fever (although the weakened body may develop various infections).

Why does a person become allergic?

It is unusual to be allergic at birth. Most allergic individuals inherit only the capacity to become allergic. They usually become sensitized to the allergen during an infection or when exposed to excessive air pollution. The mucous membranes along the respiratory tract and intestinal tract are quite efficient in keeping foreign materials from entering the body's tissues during normal health. However, inflammation caused by infections or air pollution disrupts the mucous blanket and allows penetration of the foreign proteins in an unaltered state. The body's immune system then makes antibodies which are specific for these allergens.

On later exposure to these allergens, even when the mucous membrane is intact, the immune system stimulates the release of agents by specialized cells called "mast cells" to prevent invasion by these foreign substances. These agents produce (1) edema (an abnormal accumulation of fluid), (2) congestion with increased blood flow to the local area, and (3) watery secretions. These three responses result in the allergic symptoms, which really are somewhat like "cold" symptoms.

On repeated exposure to the allergens, some patients become more and more highly sensitized. Other patients tend to do better in time. Avoidance of the allergens, if it is possible, gives much improvement.

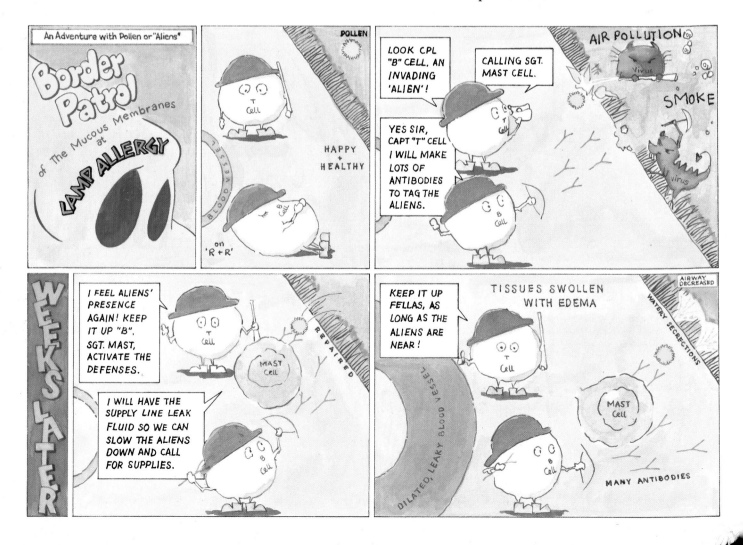

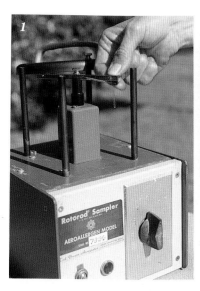

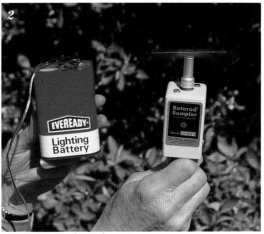

(1) Automatic pollen collector with rain-cover removed showing plastic rod lowered into position for spinning. (2) Portable field-model pollen collector in operation with rods down and spinning. A battery operated Rotorod such as this can be used to study the distance pollen travels from plants and the time of day pollen is most airborne for certain plants. The Rotorod is manufactured by Ted Brown Associates, 26338 Esperanza Drive, Los Altos Hills, CA 94022.

All about pollen

Pollens are the best studied of the allergens. The dust-like pollen grains which cause allergy are generally about three times the size of a red blood cell. Pollen grains are the small male reproductive bodies of plants, somewhat analogous to the sperm of animals, by which the female flowers (or floral parts) are fertilized.

Pollen is carried from plant to plant by insects, water, wind, gravity, and various special methods. Insect-pollinated flowers are brightly colored with perfumed nectar and large, heavy pollen. These pollens seldom get in the air. Plants that are wind-pollinated are more likely to be allergenic than plants that are insect-pollinated. Allergenic plants have inconspicuous flowers and smaller, bouyant pollen that is more plentiful in the air.

How pollen is counted

Most pollen counts were done by the gravity method prior to 1970. A glass slide was greased and placed outdoors for 24 hours in a protected manner so rain would not fall on it but air could blow over its surface and particles such as pollen would stick to it. Then the surface was stained and the pollen grains were counted with a microscope. The report stated the number of pollen grains falling on a one square centimeter area during a 24 hour period.

With the old method, very light pollens tend to remain airborne and not fall onto the slide. The new method uses a spinning rod covered with grease which strikes these small pollen grains with force when they are present in the air. The greased rod is spun through the air for one minute at 10 minute intervals.[1] The rod is retracted into a protected tunnel for the 9 minutes between spins. Every 24 hours the rod is stained and the pollen particles are counted. A known volume of air has been sampled and this count is reported as pollen grains per cubic meter of air.[1,2]

There are other methods but this is the method selected at present by the American Academy of Allergy and Immunology Pollen and Mold Committee.

The significance of pollen counts

Most plants will bloom for about 4 weeks. Some years there may be more pollen than other years and patients have more symptoms. Without treatment there is usually a high correlation between allergy symptoms and pollen counts. Therefore, allergists now compare symptom scores with pollen counts to evaluate the effectiveness of treatment programs for allergies.

How to use this book

Because of their inconspicuous flowers, allergenic plants are difficult to identify. For that reason, allergy patients can unwittingly be exposed to large numbers of their allergens. This book is designed to make it possible for allergy patients to identify and avoid the enemy (allergy plants in bloom). Elimination of all allergy plants is unrealistic and dedicated drives to accomplish this in the past have failed. However, with a little study, it is possible to avoid heavy exposure to the pollens of allergenic plants, a practical and worthwhile goal.

The plants will be presented as they appear during the year, starting with the trees which are the first to bloom.

The Pine Family

Conifers are wind-pollinated trees with very buoyant pollen that can travel hundreds of miles. The large pine pollen is the most visible and forms a yellow dust on dark objects when the trees are in bloom.[3] Even though pine pollen is carried by wind and abundant in most parts of the continent, it is seldom an important allergen. The allergenic components of the pine pollen just do not evoke a strong allergic response. There have been, however, a few rare cases of pine pollen allergy. The abundantly visible but innocuous pollen appears as early as January in southern areas and as late as May or June in northern mountains.

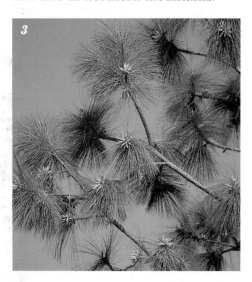

The male flowers[4] have powdery yellow pollen on their surface and occur in clusters of purplish, spindle-shaped cones. The female flowers[5] produce multiple scales in the form of a cone. Male and female flowers are at tips of separate tree branches. Spruce, fir, hemlock, larch and the true cedars (cedar of Lebanon and deodar cedar, neither being native to America) have large, non-allergenic pollen similar to that of

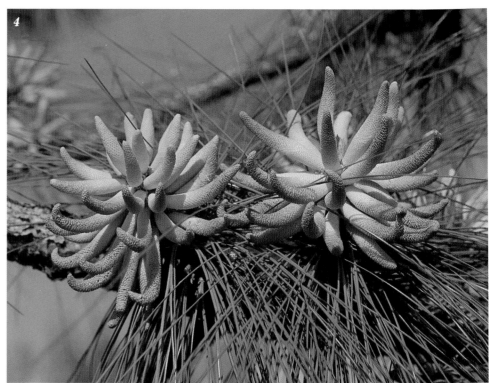

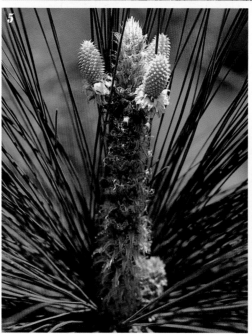

(3) Blooming long-leaf pine. (4) Long-leaf pine, male flowers. (5) Female flowers developing into cones. (6) Pollen on car. The tree reflected in the car hood is not blooming, nor are any trees nearby. This demonstrates the abundance of pollen in the air from a variety of sources. Pine pollen is the pollen most frequently noticed with the naked eye because it is larger than most other pollens.

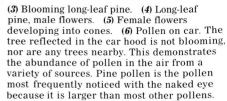

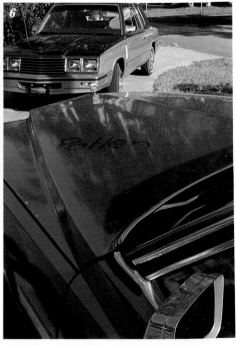

the pines. In areas where pine is common, the pollen's presence is readily noticed, particularly by scrupulous housekeepers. A yellow dust film[6] settles on everything and illustrates how plentiful pollen is in our environment.

Juniper/Cypress and Sequoia Families

Mountain (Mexican) juniper, white and red cedars (junipers),[7] Arizona cypress, Monterey cypress, bald cypress, and sequoia are all somewhat related and have more toxic pollen than the pines. The pollen is very buoyant and is smaller than pine pollen. There is a lot of cross-reactivity* among this group. For instance, people allergic to eastern white cedar often develop symptoms when traveling to areas where the eastern white cedar does not grow. Exposure to a related cypress can trigger an allergic reaction to the antigens** or allergens of its pollen in a person sensitive to eastern white cedar.

In Texas, where the mountain cedar *(Juniperus ashei;* syn: *J. mexicana;* syn: *J. sabinoides)* grows like a weed in overgrazed grasslands, this allergenic tree has become a prominent problem. In the far South, junipers bloom in January. The Bermuda juniper *(J. bermudiana)* is nearly the only hay fever plant in Bermuda, blooming in March and April. In western Texas, Arizona, and parts of California, the Pinchot juniper blooms from September through November and not in the spring.

Most of the junipers have separate male and female plants. The male flowers are found in tiny cones[8] at the branch tips, and their pollen will appear as smoke[9] in the air if the branch is physically disturbed.

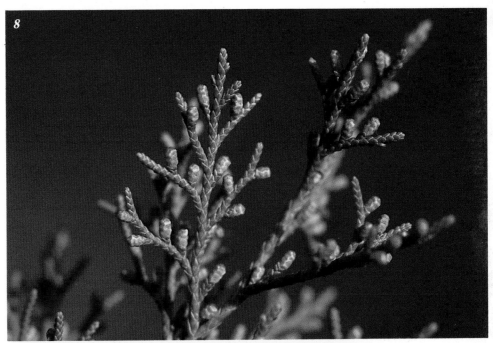

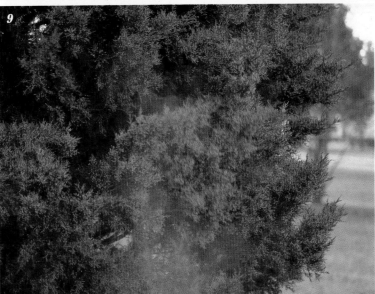

(7) Juniper tree *(Juniperus silicicola).* (8) Juniper male "flowers" (small cones) close-up. (9) Juniper male tree with pollen "smoking" from a disturbed branch.

*Cross-reactive: evoking a response to one pollen or allergen as though it was another similar pollen or allergen to which one has become sensitized.

**Antigens: substances that provoke immune responses when introduced to tissues or the blood stream. Allergens are antigens. Antigen is a broader concept including substances such as bacteria, endotoxins, viruses, etc. The terms antigen and allergen can be used interchangeably for the allergic reaction provokers.

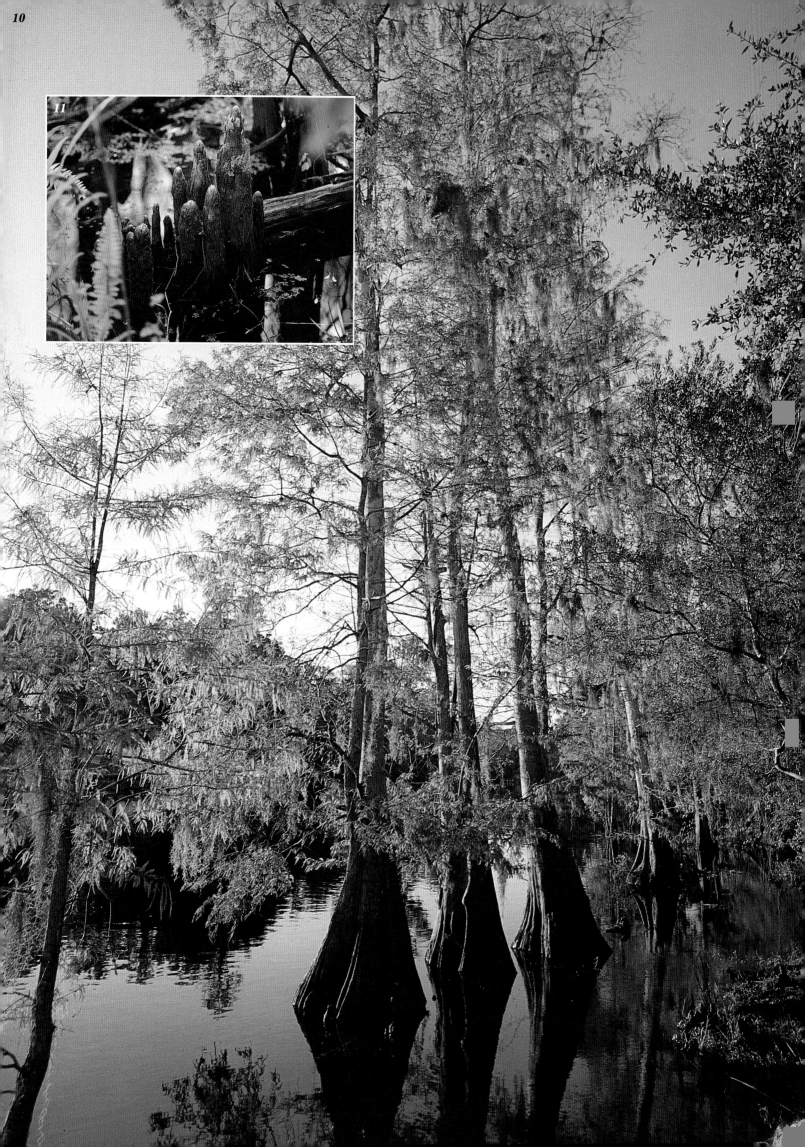

11

0) Bald cypress
owing fluted base of
unks in fresh water.
1) Cypress "knees"
oot projections).

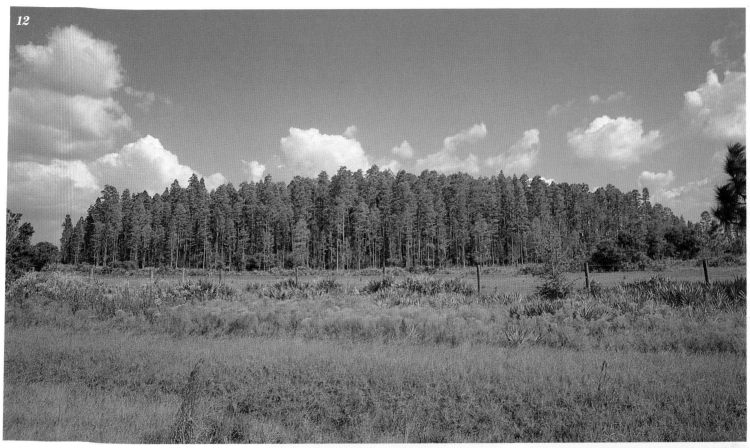

Juniper/Cypress and Sequoia Families *(continued)*

The female trees produce the berry-like fruits. A juniper with berries will not produce pollen. Numerous homes have landscaping with small junipers near doorways, and exposure to their pollen can be heavy.

Close relatives and cross-reactors with the junipers, the cypresses[12] have inconspicuous male and female cone-like flowers on the same tree but on different twigs.

If Chinese patients have allergic symptoms during the tree season, they most often are sensitive to cedars, cypress, and junipers.

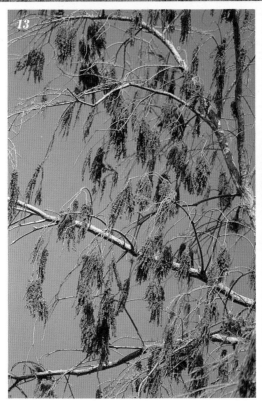

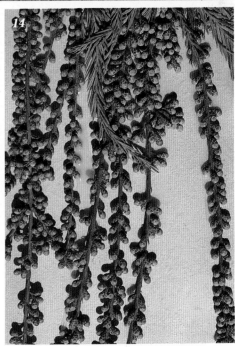

(12) Bald cypress dome. *(13)* Bald cypress tree with leaves off and with drooping tassels. *(14)* Bald cypress (*Taxodium distichum*) male tassels of conelets close-up.

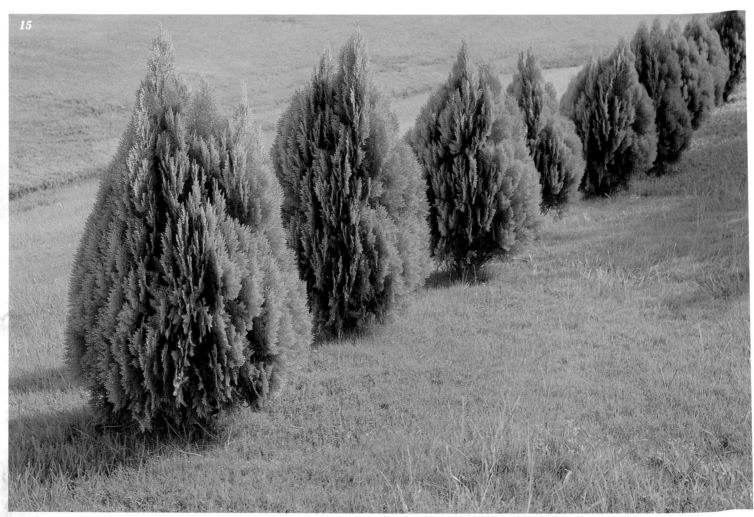

15

(15)Arborvitae. (16) Arborvitae with flower formation at tips of scale-like leaves. Later this becomes brown and inconspicuous.

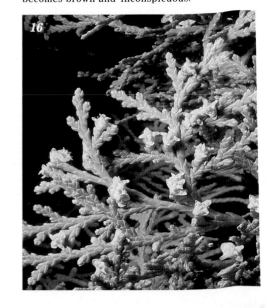

16

Juniper/Cypress and Sequoia Families *(continued)*

The coast redwood *(Sequoia)*, Japanese cedar *(Cryptomeria)*, and bald cypress *(Taxodium)* have slightly different antigenic characteristics than the junipers and cypresses, but all are wind-pollinated and potentially allergenic. *Sequoia* and bald cypress[10-14] grow mainly in unpopulated areas, parks, and wildlife preservations. Japanese cedar *(Cryptomeria)* is planted for landscaping and wind-breaks in Hawaii and the west coast of the U.S. The bald cypress and the larch are two conifers that are deciduous; that is, their needles fall off completely in the late fall. The male flowers of bald cypress are conelets on long, drooping tassels;[13,14] the female flowers develop into small, woody cones on separate branches.

Arborvitae[15] *(Platycladus* or *Thuja)* is a common ornamental evergreen that blooms with male and female flowers[16] on different branches at the tips of scale-like leaves, later than junipers, in March and April.

Ginkgo

Native to China, the ginkgo,[17] also called the maidenhair tree, is one of the more primitive trees. Male and female flowers are found on separate trees. The female trees are shunned as ornamentals because the putrid-smelling fruits attract insects, but male trees, which are capable of shedding much pollen, are frequently planted. Ginkgo has been widely planted throughout the United States. Although large amounts of its pollen can get into the air, sensitivity to this plant has not been well studied.

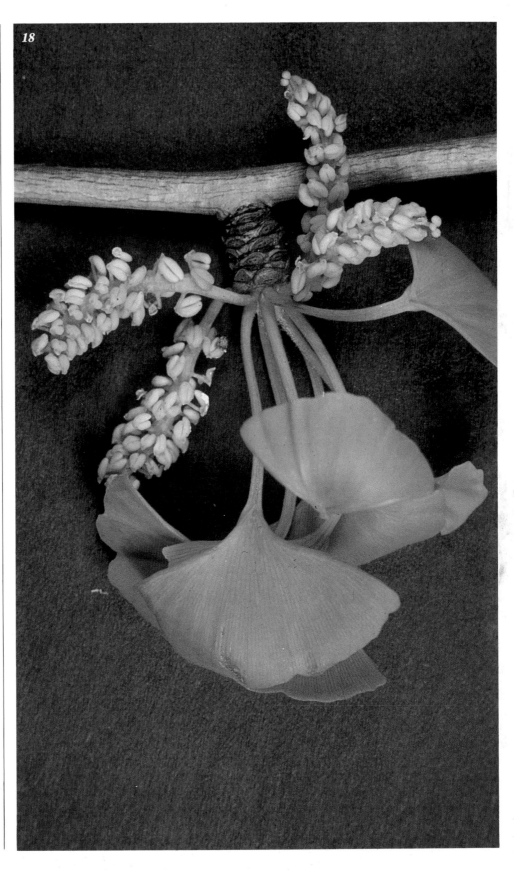

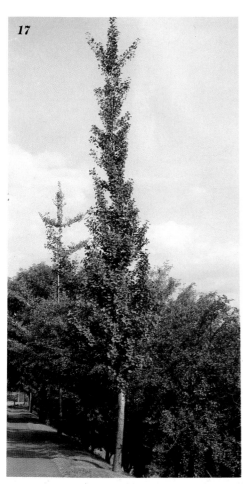

(**17**) Young ginkgo. (**18**) Ginkgo close-up of male bloom. Different sexes are on separate trees.

ANGIOSPERMS

SEED-BEARING PLANTS

Dicotyledons: plants having two seed-leaves on baby plants

The Maple Family

Box elder *(Acer negundo),*[20] a fast growing tree common in the Midwest, is the most potent member of the maple family. This tree breaks the rule advising one to avoid plants having three-parted compound leaves, since box elder does not have contact irritants like poison ivy. Its blooms appear before the leaves unfold, in January and February in southernmost areas and in April and May in northeastern and mid-western states. Although related to box elder, the other maples[19] cause fewer allergy problems.

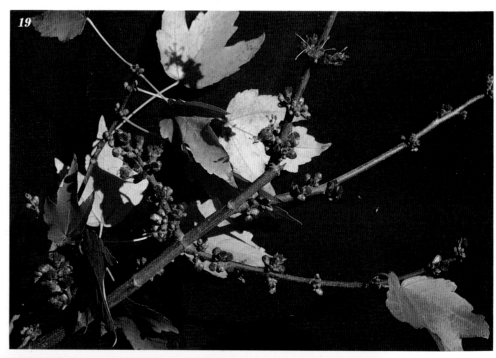

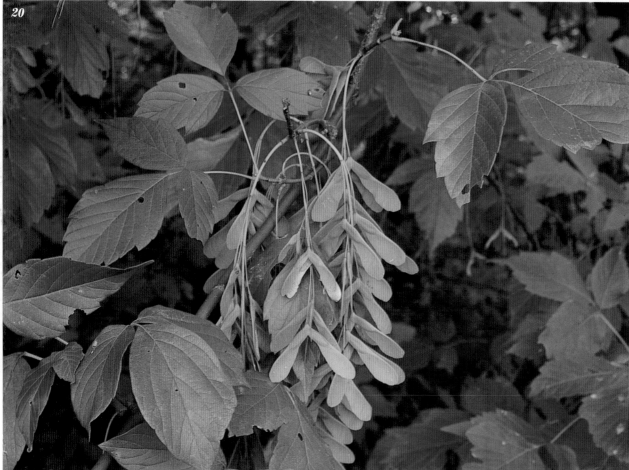

(*19*) Maple *(Acer)* in bloom before new leaves appear, but with some old leaves. (*20*) Box elder *(Acer negundo)* with samaras (winged fruits).

The Willow/Poplar Family

Willows have male and female flowers on different trees and bloom in March and April. They are mainly insect-pollinated, but the pollen, which is small and numerous, is also transported by wind. It is not a strong allergen. The pussy willow (Salix discolor) produces its catkins* long before the leaves appear, but it is of no allergic significance. The color and nectar of the flowers attract insects, and there is less airborne pollen than is produced by the less showy willows. Black willow (S. nigra)[23] is common throughout the eastern states along streams and lakes, and its catkins open after the narrow, lance-shaped leaves are fully extended.

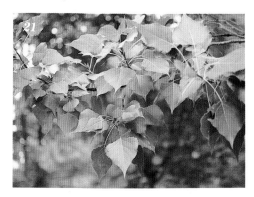

The poplars, aspens and cottonwoods are entirely wind-pollinated. They have drooping catkins with male and female flowers on separate trees. The eastern cottonwood (Populus deltoides)[21] is most prevalent along streams of midwestern and eastern states. The balsam poplar and aspen are prevalent in Canada, the Rockies, and Alaska. These mildly allergenic trees bloom in April and May. Many of the ornamental poplars are sterile hybrids with showy catkins which produce no pollen, and these trees are ideal to grow for people suffering from allergies.

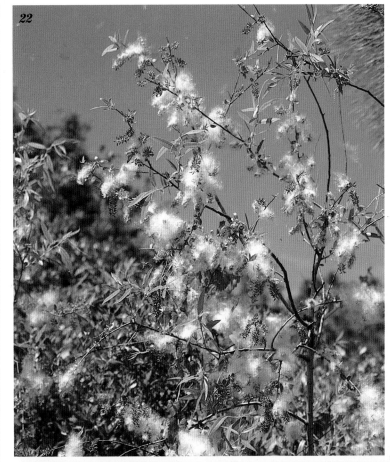

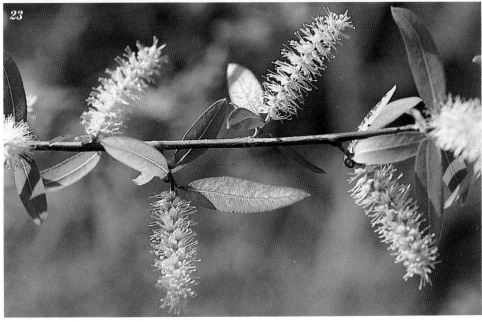

*Catkins: elongated spike-like clusters of tiny flowers. Male catkins are usually long and drooping, the female short and upright.

(21) Eastern cottonwood (Populus deltoides). (22) Willow with seeds. The seeds of poplars and willows, with their white fluffy "parachutes," are very visible and often blamed for any allergy symptoms suffered at the time the seeds appear. These allergy symptoms are most likely caused by other less visible allergens in the air. (23) Willow flowers. Willows are pollinated by insects and also by the wind.

Dicots

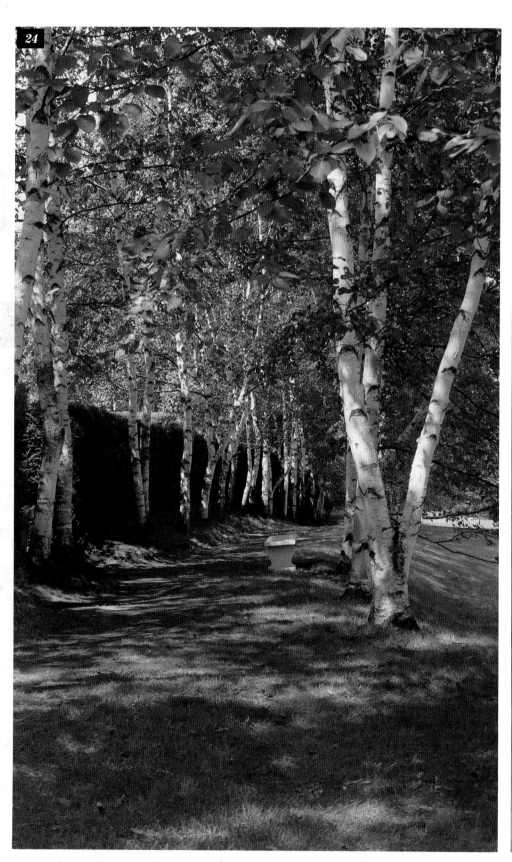

The Birch Family

Birch *(Betula)* trees bloom generously in the eastern states in April and May. Pollen falls from hanging catkins which formed the previous year. Most birches have very scaly bark. The gray[25] · and white birches[24] bloom in April in the northeastern states, across Canada, and into Alaska. The yellow birch and sweet birch[26] are found in the Appalachian Mountain region and upper Midwest. The river birch *(B. nigra)*[25] grows along streams in the southeastern states and blooms from March to mid-April.

Alders *(Alnus)*[27] are found in the eastern United States and in the Pacific Northwest. They have drooping male catkins[28] and upright female catkins persisting from the previous year, and they produce much pollen from February through April before the leaves appear. Many people have allergic reactions to this pollen.

The hornbeams *(Carpinus)*, hophornbeams *(Ostrya)*[29] and hazels *(Corylus)* are related to the birches and alders and cross-react with them. They have double-toothed leaves (as do birches, alders and elms) and dangling male and female catkins. Hornbeams grow in the eastern U.S. Hazel ranges from the East to Wyoming.

(**24**) White birch trees. (**25**) Dried specimens: top is gray birch *(Betula populifolia)*, bottom is river birch *(Betula nigra)*. (**26**) Sweet birch *(Betula lenta)*. (**27**) Alder leaves. (**28**) Alder *(Alnus serrulata)* with blooming catkins, before leaves emerge. (**29**) Hophornbeam with fruits. *(Ostrya virginiana)*.

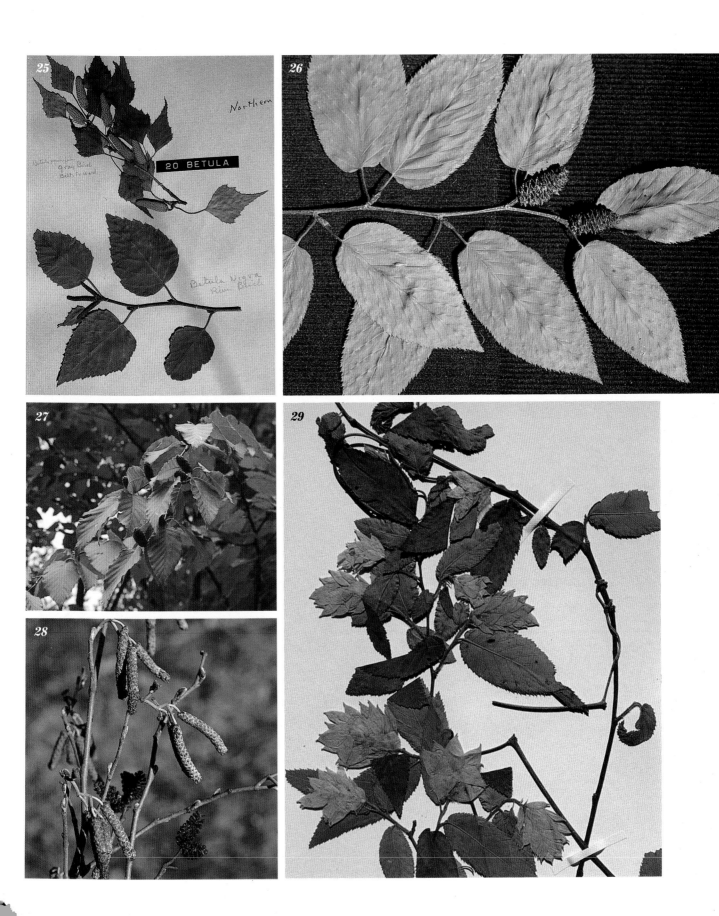

Dicots

The Elm Family[30]

The American elm (*Ulmus americana*) is widespread through the eastern and midwestern states. It blooms[32] early in February in the South and in March and April in the North with small inconspicuous flowers before the leaves appear. It is moderately strongly allergenic. A fungus known as Dutch elm disease[30] has attacked American elms since 1930 and tragically decreased their numbers. The rock elm (*U. thomasii*) ranges from the midwestern to northeastern states, and the winged elm (*U. alata*) is found in the southern states. Both of these elms bloom in the spring. The cedar elm (*U. crassifolia*) and September elm (*U. serotina*) grow mainly in southern states. They bloom in the fall from August to October and produce strong allergens. Elm flowers are bisexual, each flower having both male and female parts.

Hackberries[33] and sugarberries (*Celtis*) grow southward and eastward from Illinois and bloom in April as their leaves unfold. These are important allergenic trees in Oklahoma and Texas, but are not very prevalent in other areas.

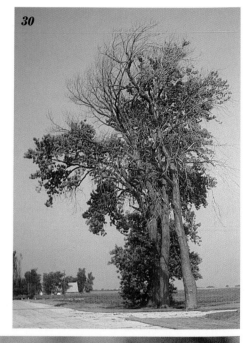

(**30**) American elm which has been killed by Dutch elm disease. (**31**) Elm leaves. Siberian elm (*Ulmus pumila*), top, and slippery elm (*Ulmus rubra*), bottom. (**32**) Elm (*Ulmus americana*) in bloom before leaves appear. (**33**) Hackberry.

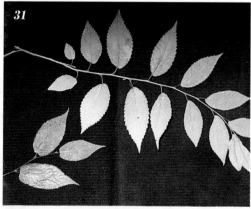

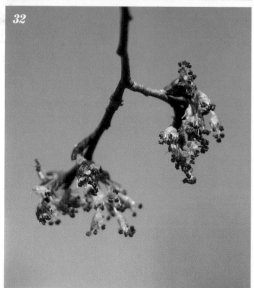

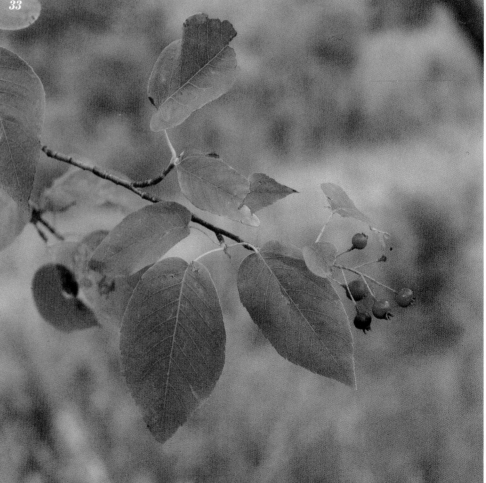

The Mulberry Family

The mulberry family includes the white and red mulberries *(Morus alba* and *M. rubra)*,[35] the paper mulberry *(Broussonetia)*[34] and the osage orange or hedge plant *(Maclura)*. The paper mulberry and hedge plant are important allergenic plants which bloom in April and May. The male catkins are present just before the leaves appear.[35] The paper mulberry was planted widely in southern states, initially to develop a silkworm industry. Male and female flowers are on separate plants. The osage orange was planted as a hedge and its wood used for fence posts. It is present in the lower Midwest and South.

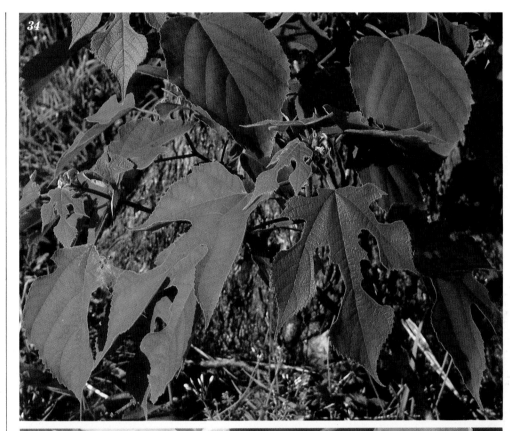

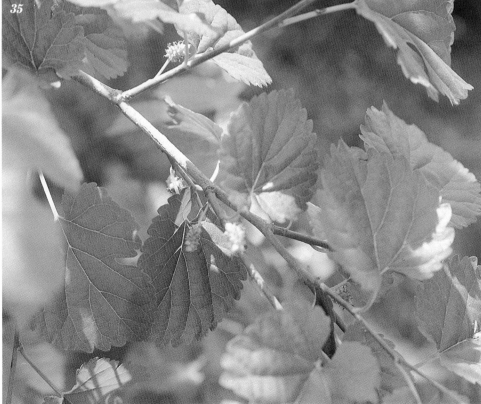

(*34*) Paper mulberry *(Broussonetia papyrifera)*.
(*35*) White mulberry *(Morus alba)* with catkins and early spring leaves.

The Beech/Oak Family

While the European beeches cause allergies, the American species is not an important problem. The related chestnuts and tanoaks are insect-pollinated.

The oaks *(Quercus)*[36-41] shed more pollen than all other plants where the trees are abundant. Oaks are present in all states except Alaska and Hawaii, and they are very prevalent in the southeastern and southwestern states. They are important causes of allergies.

The identification of oaks is very difficult because of their tendency to hybridize (interbreed). The drooping male catkins release pollen in February and March in the South and April and May in northern states. Often there are several species, with one blooming after another to give a prolonged period of pollen release. The antigens cross-react with each other but may also be uniquely different.

Thus, it is important to skin test for the species of oaks from the region in which the patient resides. There are about 60 species native to the U.S., and these are artificially divided into red and white oak groups.

The red oaks have bristle-tips on the leaves and dark bark. Their acorns are bitter and inedible, have yellow meat, hairs inside the

---

(36) Live oak tree. (37) Live oak (*Quercus virginiana*) with catkin blooms. (38) Water oak (*Quercus nigra*) in bloom. (39) Myrtle oak (*Quercus myrtifolia*) in heavy bloom.

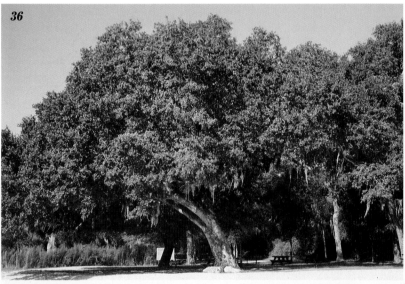

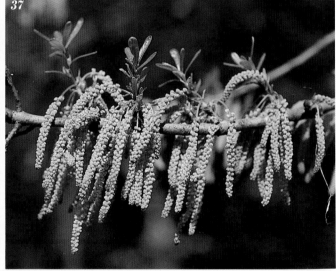

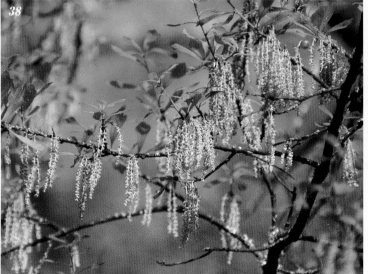

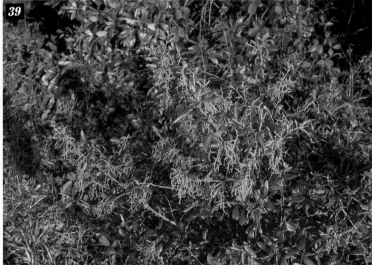

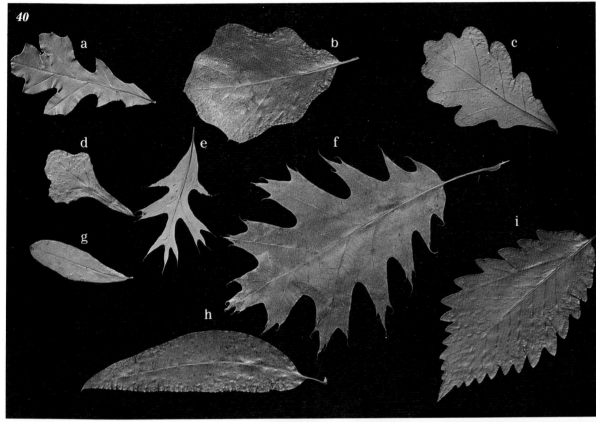

40

(40) a. Overcup oak (*Q. lyrata*)
　　　b. Blackjack oak
　　　　(*Q. marilandica*)
　　　c. White oak (*Q. alba*)
　　　d. Water oak (*Q. nigra*)
　　　e Turkey oak (*Q. laevis*)
　　　f. Red oak (*Q. falcata*)
　　　g. Live oak (*Q. virginiana*)
　　　h. Willow oak (*Q. phellos*)
　　　i. Chestnut oak (*Q. prinus*)

(41) White oak with acorns.

shells, and require two years for maturation. The white oaks do not have bristle-tipped leaves, and their bark is lighter in color. Their acorns develop in one year. The meat is white, sweet, and edible, and the shells are usually hairless inside. There are some species in the western states that have traits of both white and red oaks. The oaks can be further divided into those with lobed leaves, those with toothed or wavy leaves, and those with plain or smooth leaf margins.[40]

Some oaks do not shed their leaves in the fall but drop them as the new foliage appears in the spring. These oaks are referred to as evergreen. Examples of evergreen oaks include the live oaks, myrtle oak, and California scrub oak. Laurel oak sheds its leaves so late in the spring that it is referred to as "semi-evergreen."

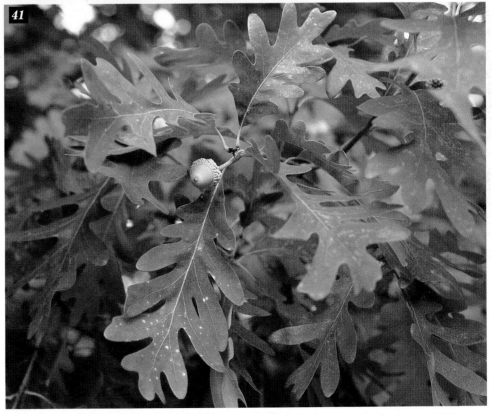

41

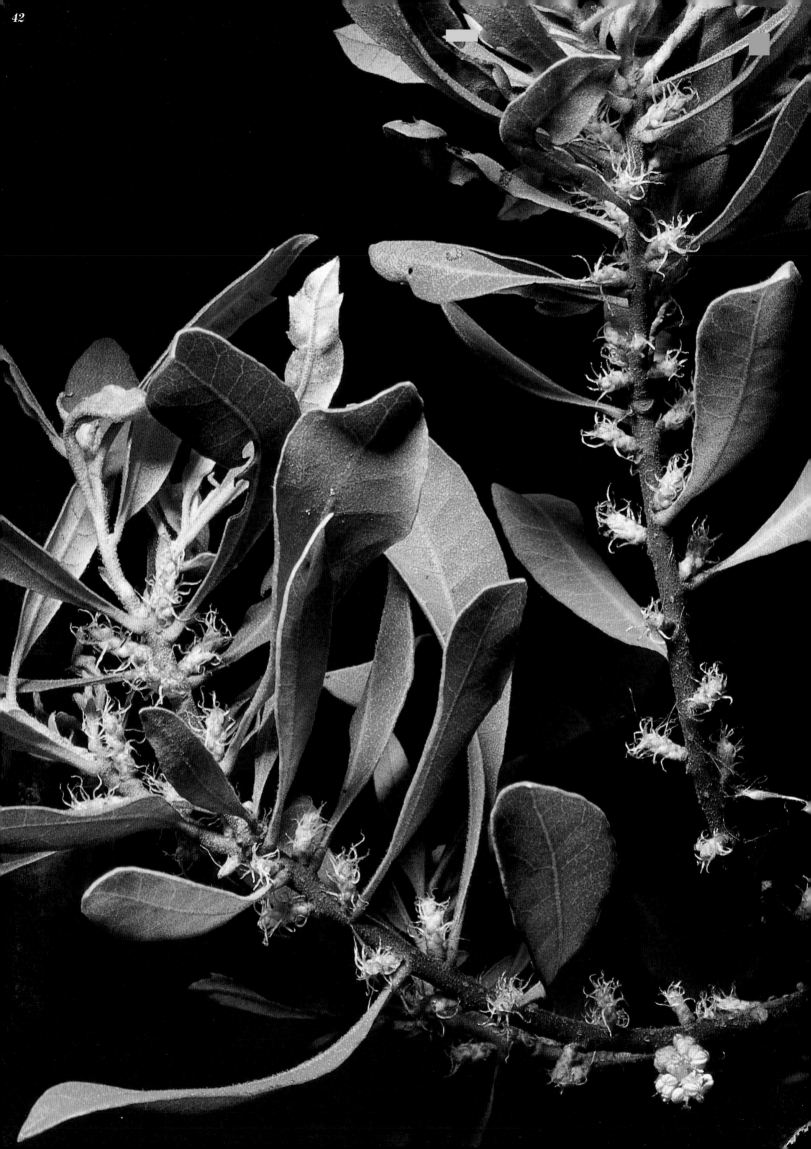

Dicots

The Bayberry Family

Bayberries or wax myrtles *(Myrica)*[42-44] are shrubs or small trees of the coastal plain of the Atlantic and Gulf states and California. They produce small catkins at the base of the leaves. The male and female flowers[42,43] are found on separate trees of the eastern species. However, on the California wax myrtle the two sexes are borne on the same plant. The leaves have a pleasant aroma when crushed and are coated with glandular dots below.[43] The northern bayberry is deciduous (drops its leaves in the fall) while the other species are evergreen. The southern bayberry blooms in February and March, and the northern bayberry blooms in April and May.

The sweet fern *(Comptonia)*, a relative, is not a fern but a shrub with fern-like leaves that are also aromatic. It grows in Canada and the northeastern U.S. Bayberry and sweet fern are moderately strongly allergenic plants.

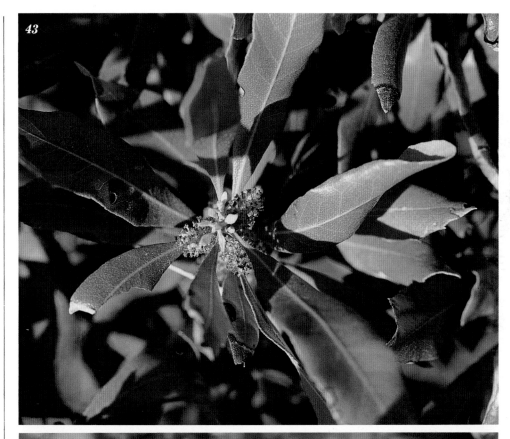

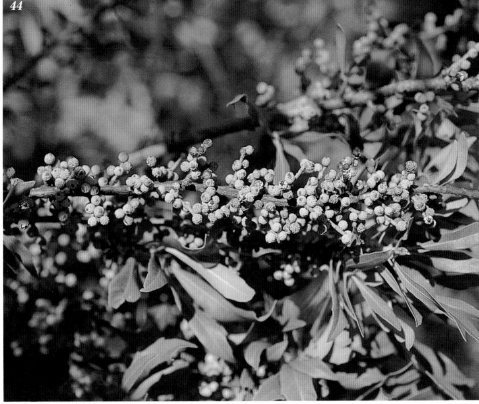

(42) Bayberry (*Myrica cerifera*). Female with bloom. **(43)** Male bayberry (*M. cerifera*) with bloom. **(44)** Female bayberry (*M. cerifera*) with waxy blue-green fruits.

Australian Pine

Beefwood or Australian pines *(Casuarina)*[45-47] are not true pines (and they are not even conifers), showing that common names can be misleading. They are native to tropical Asia and Australia and were brought to Florida and California for use as windbreaks. In Florida, they were an unfortunate introduction. They grow rapidly and aggressively and shade out the desirable native plants which help prevent beach erosion with their more extensive root systems. Australian pines have shallow roots and are often blown over by strong winds.[46]

The male blooms are at the tips of branches which look like needles. The true leaves are tiny and scale-like, in rings or whorls at the joints of the green "needles." When in bloom, the trees appear rusty, bearing pollen at the tips of all the drooping, needle-like twigs. Both male and female flowers are found on the same trees. The female flowers are clustered balls on the sides of the twigs near the tips of the branches. Australian pines are entirely wind-pollinated and bloom in the spring and the fall. The pollen has moderately strong antigens.

Australian pines are subtropical. *Casuarina cunninghamiana* tolerates cold a little better than *Casuarina equisetifolia*, but neither can survive temperatures below 28 degrees for long periods. The scalybark beefwood *(C. cristata)* spreads from suckers and is not tolerant of salt spray. This species has not been widely planted.

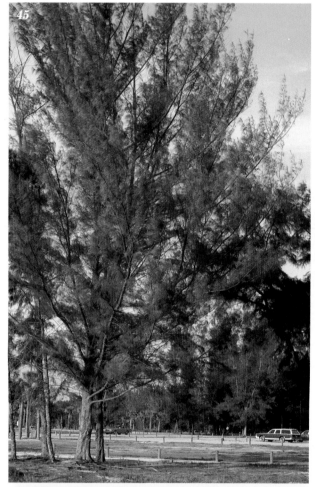

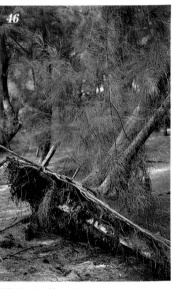

(45) Australian pine trees preventing growth of ground cover.
(46) Australian pine tree tipped over because of shallow root system.
(47) Australian pine blooms, male at tips and female closer to woody branch. The green "needles" are twigs and the leaves are the tiny, paler green scales at each joint.

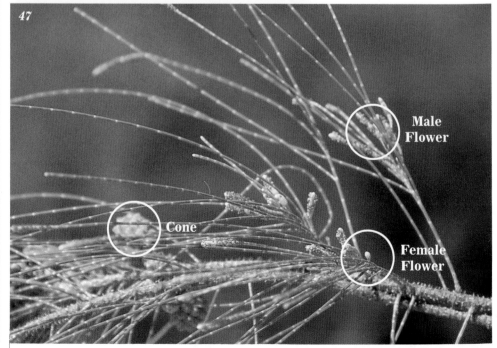

Male Flower

Cone

Female Flower

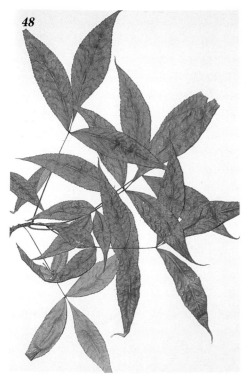

48

(48) The leaves of ash (*Fraxinus*). (49) Ash blooms. The new leaves are just starting to develop. (50) *Ligustrum* with flowers at tip of branch. Clipping will prevent bloom from forming. Note glossy leaves.

The Olive Family

The ashes *(Fraxinus)*[48] are very widespread trees found in all of the U.S. except the Rockies. They grow well on a variety of sites, including hillsides, but they are most often found in low, moist or wet areas. Their leaves are compound, being formed by 5 to 9 sharp-pointed leaflets with short stems. The flowers[49] appear before the leaves, in February and March in the South and May in the North. In most species, there are separate male and female trees. The fruits or seeds resemble maple seeds, with their papery wings, and they appear in the summer in clusters. Ashes are entirely wind-pollinated, and the pollen is moderately allergenic. Mountain ash *(Sorbus)* is not related. It belongs to the rose family and is entirely insect-pollinated.

The olive trees of the Mediterranean area are related to ashes and were introduced into the southwestern states and southern Florida. Olives are partly wind-pollinated and are strongly allergenic in the Mediterranean and the southwestern U.S.

Ligustrum, or privet, belongs to the olive family and is an evergreen with glossy leaves. It is used in landscaping and as a hedge. It is insect-pollinated, with white clusters of flowers[50] at the tips of branches from June through September. The flowers have an odor of fresh fish. Some of the pollen escapes into the air for short distances. Some patients' symptoms have been correlated with exposure to *Ligustrum* and positive skin tests, but it is not an important allergenic plant. Frequent clipping of the hedge can significantly reduce the blooms.

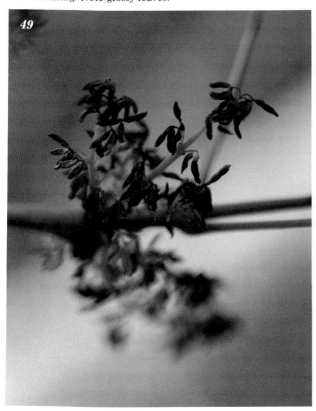

49

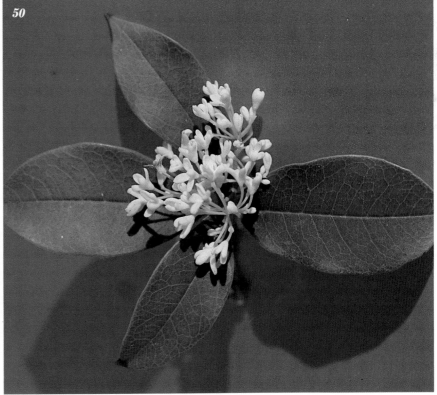

50

The Pecan/Walnut Family

Pecans and walnuts[51] have compound leaves with lance-shaped leaflets. Pecans have 11 to 17 such leaflets, and walnuts have 12 to 24 per leaf. The male catkins[52] are multiple, long, and drooping. The female bloom is very short, inconspicuous and upright. Both male and female flowers are on the same tree, but in different sites.

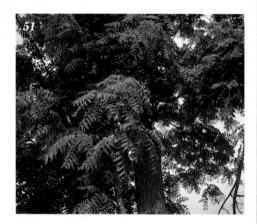

Black walnut is found in the midwestern to mideastern states. The English walnut is not native but it is commercially grown in California and causes allergy there. Walnuts bloom in April and May. The pecan grows and is cultivated from Texas to the Southeast and blooms from March to May, causing local allergy problems.

There are many species of hickories[53] that grow throughout the eastern U.S. and Texas. These trees have compound leaves resembling those of the pecan, but with fewer leaflets (3 to 13). Their flowering pattern and season is also similar to the pecan.

The pollen of all these trees is large and does not travel far. However, in areas where the trees are cultivated commercially, heavy exposure to the pollen can cause allergy symptoms.

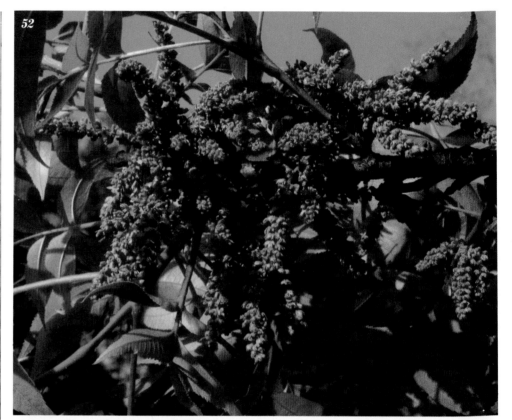

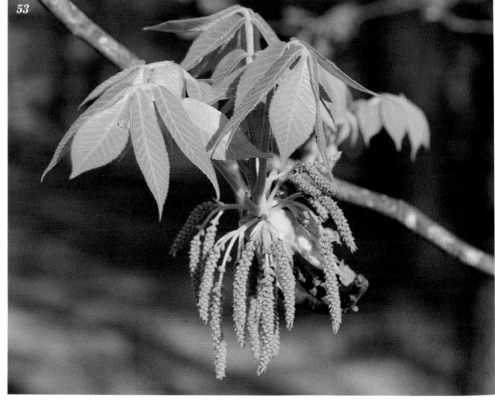

(51) Walnut tree. (52) Pecan bloom. (53) Hickory bloom.

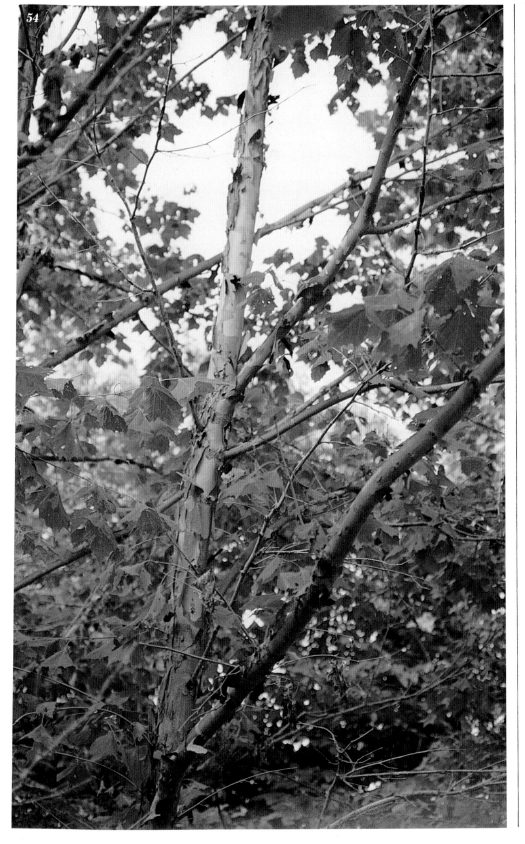

Sycamore

The sycamore or planetree *(Platanus)*[54] is a beautiful, large tree with patchy, peeling bark of varying hues of white, gray, green and brown. Its very large leaves resemble overgenerous maple leaves. Male and female flowers are found on the same tree, and in the spring they appear among the new leaves in dense clusters shaped like small balls. The fruits are bright green balls, one inch in diameter, which turn yellowish-brown at maturity. The pollen is small, wind-borne, and moderately allergenic. Sycamores are found throughout the eastern states and are common as ornamental street trees in cities.

There is a western sycamore in the California-Arizona region. The western blooming season is only two to three weeks long in April and May.

(54) Young sycamore tree *(Platanus)*. Note the peeling bark of multiple hues. **(55)** The large leaves of sycamore.

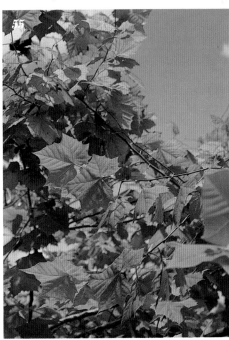

The Sweetgum/Witch Hazel Family

Sweetgum (*Liquidambar*),[56] a large tree, has star-shaped leaves and flowers, in balls, which release pollen in April and May. The pollen is large, but is nevertheless wind-borne. Witch hazel (*Hamamelis*),[57] a relative, is more of a shrub. It has smaller pollen and blooms in the fall (November and December). When the fruits mature, the seeds are forcibly ejected, shooting out quite a distance. Sweetgum and witch hazel are eastern plants and are only mildly allergenic.

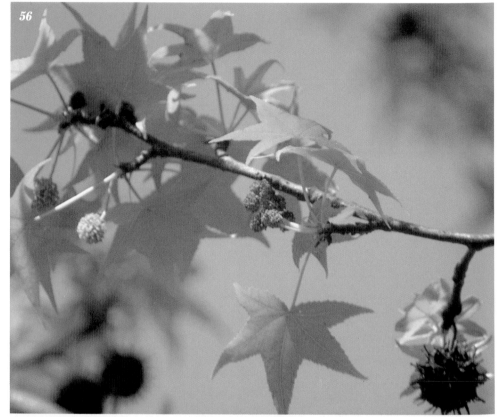

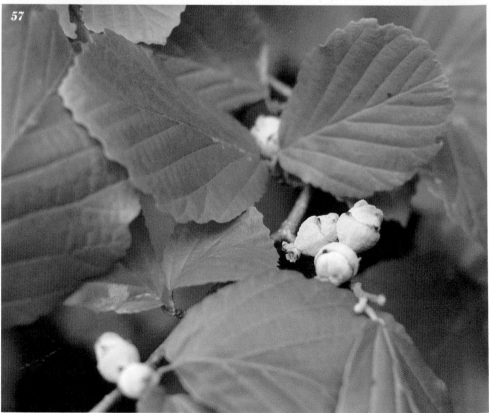

(**56**) Sweetgum (*Liquidambar*) with fresh bloom and the fruit of the previous year. (**57**) Witch hazel with fruit.

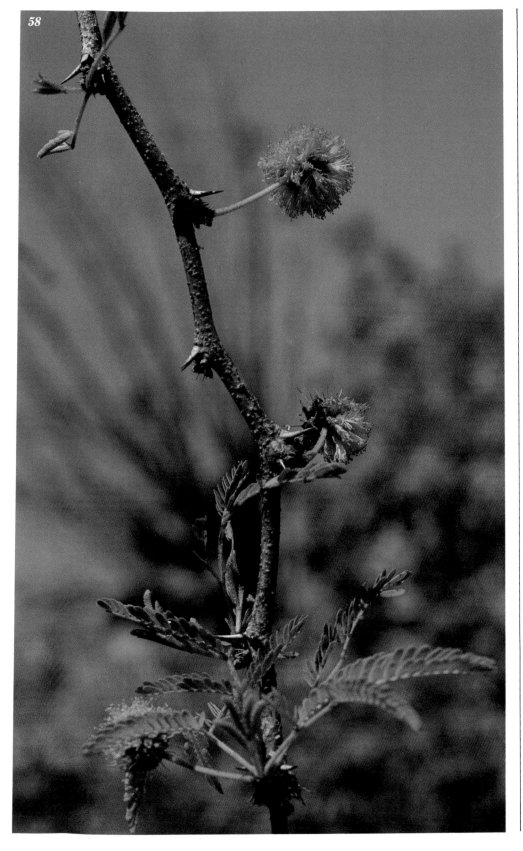

58

The Legume Family

Mesquite *(Prosopis)*[59] is partially insect-pollinated, but it has been reported to cause allergy problems in Texas, New Mexico, southeastern California, and Hawaii from May through July. Its leaves are doubly compound, and its greenish-white flowers are borne on two-inch long, cylindrical spikes. The wood is very popular for barbeques, but there have been no reports of allergy to the smoke. Acacia[58] is widely planted as an ornamental. It blooms from January through October in California and is reported to cause allergy problems there even though it is insect-pollinated. Acacia gum, also called gum arabic, is used in sizing, hair dressings, and as a thickening agent in many foods and pharmaceuticals. In these forms it can cause symptoms from inhalation of the dried powder.

---

(58) Sweet acacia (*Acacia farnesiana*) is mainly insect-pollinated, but it commonly grows along roadways in California and the heavy traffic whirls the acacia pollen into the air.
(59) Mesquite (*Prosopis*). Note compound leaves and cylindrical flower spikes (dried specimen).

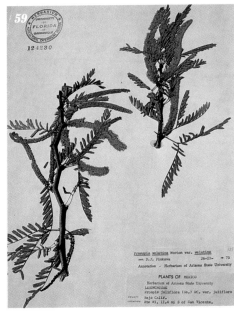

The Linden Family

Although linden *(Tilia)*[60] is considered highly allergenic in some European areas, it is not in this country. This lack of allergenic activity may be related to its insect-pollination here. Jute *(Corchorus)*, a relative, is not a pollen problem but its fibers cause inhalant allergy. The fibers are used in rope, carpet and upholstery backings.

(60) Linden *(Tilia)* heavy with fruits on stems emerging from the undersides of leaf-like bracts. **(61)** Eucalyptus with flower buds.

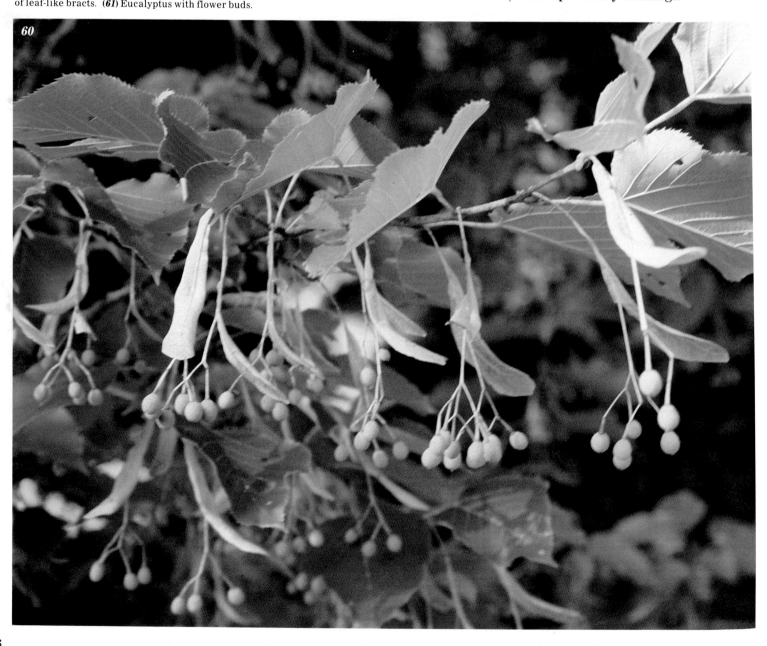

Melaleuca

The cajeput or punk tree (*Melaleuca*) is native to Australia. Its pollen is not a significant allergen, contrary to popular belief. Recent bronchial challenge tests and a number of other tests failed to elicit an allergic response in individuals who thought they had allergies to this plant (Dr. R. F. Lockey). Other, less conspicuous, plants that bloom at the same time as the punk tree may have caused the allergies. *Melaleuca* is not pictured in this book to avoid perpetuating the myth that it is a cause of allergy problems.

Citrus

Citrus flowers are insect-pollinated and virtually no pollen gets into the air. Accordingly, citrus does not cause allergy problems except by ingestion of the fruit or contact with its sap.

Eucalyptus

Eucalyptus[61] has been reported to occasionally cause allergy problems in California and Hawaii. In Florida, eucalyptus trees appear to be mainly insect-pollinated, although the pollen is sometimes found in air surveys.

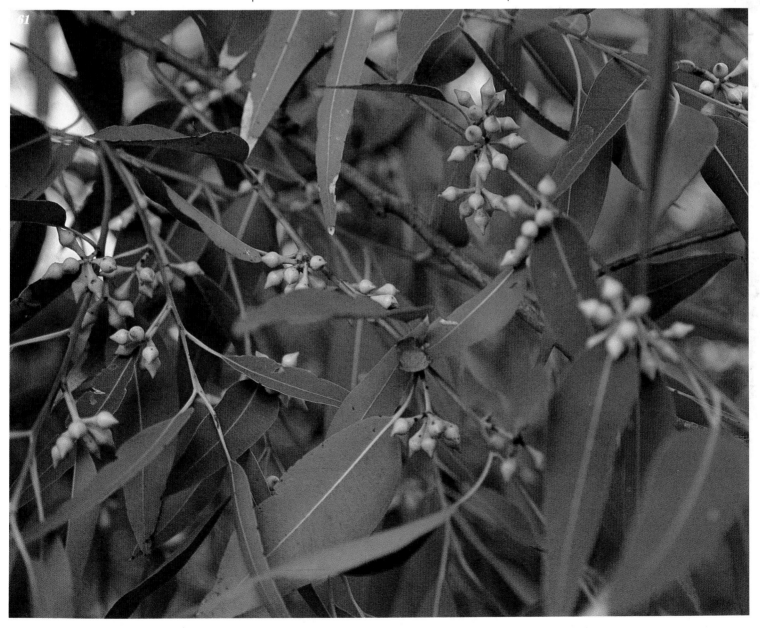

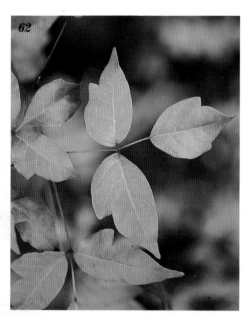

(62) Poison ivy: beware of "leaves of three."

(63) Poison ivy bloom (enlarged). **(64)** Mango in bloom. Contact with mango sap or the juice from the skin of the mango fruit can give a sensitive person a rash just like poison ivy.

Plants Causing Rashes

Poison ivy[62,63] causes a skin reaction on sensitive people which is delayed for 24 to 48 hours following contact with the plant. This reaction will appear as a red swollen area followed by water blisters and intense itching which may remain for a full week or longer. An oleoresin in the plant's sap is the allergen. Similar substances are present in poison oak, pistachio *(Pistacia)*, poison sumac, mango *(Mangifera indica)*,[64] cashew *(Anacardium occidentale)*, Brazilian pepper *(Schinus terebinthifolius)*,[65] and poisonwood *(Metopium toxiferum)*. All of these plants are members of the same family. Washing immediately after contact will prevent pain, suffering, and financial woes. Avoidance of these plants is the simple and practical way to prevent poison ivy rashes. Injection therapy can have complications and is of doubtful value.

Other allergenic plants giving delayed contact rashes are ragweed, marsh-elder, chrysanthemum, marigold, dog fennel, aster, feverfew,[68] buttercup, aloe, agave, agrimony,[66] tung nut, manchineel, and castor bean.[67]

Often confused with poison ivy rashes is photodermatitis. Photodermatitis is a rash caused by exposure to sunlight following skin contact with any one of a large number of plants. Celery, citrus, and plants of the composite family can cause photodermatitis.

Other rashes confused with poison ivy are caused by plants having chemically irritating sap. This is not allergy. Most of the spurge *(Euphorbia)* plants have irritating sap. (See Spurge section, page 57.)

Plants with stinging hairs such as nettles *(Urtica)*, horse nettle *(Solanum carolinense)* and tread softly *(Cnidoscolus stimulosus)*,[69] give a rash that can itch and look like hives and is often assumed to be an allergic reaction but is not.

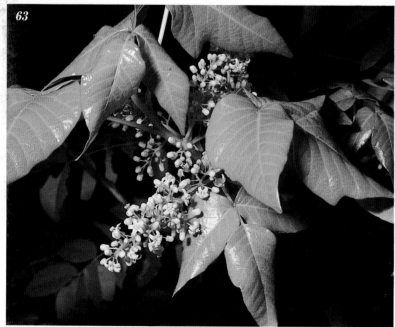

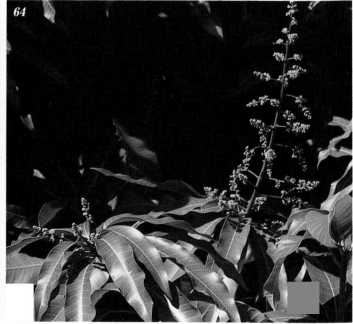

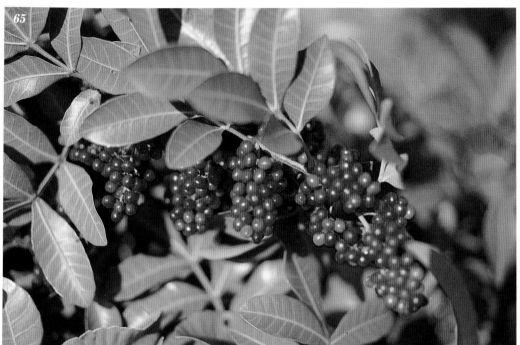

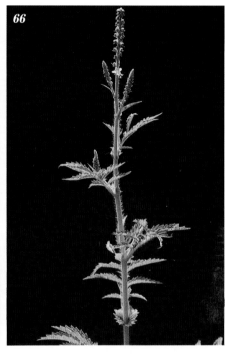

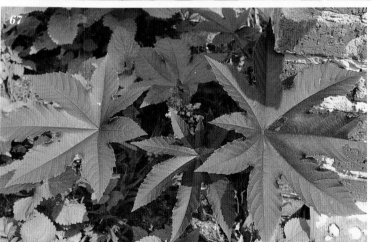

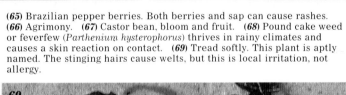

(65) Brazilian pepper berries. Both berries and sap can cause rashes. (66) Agrimony. (67) Castor bean, bloom and fruit. (68) Pound cake weed or feverfew (*Parthenium hysterophorus*) thrives in rainy climates and causes a skin reaction on contact. (69) Tread softly. This plant is aptly named. The stinging hairs cause welts, but this is local irritation, not allergy.

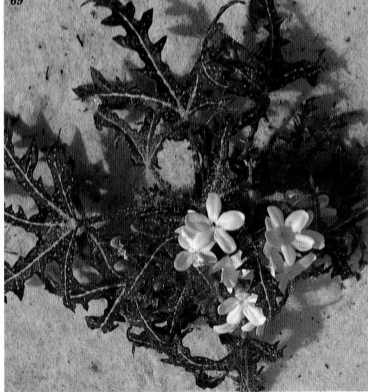

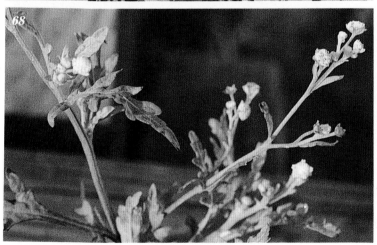

ANGIOSPERMS

SEED-BEARING PLANTS

 Monocotyledons:
Plants having single
seed leaves on
baby plants

Monocots include grasses and palms, among which are found the most important plants for man's existence. Economically important grasses include corn, wheat, rice, oats, sugar cane, and bamboo, to mention a few of the many grasses cultivated by man.

The Palm Family

The palm family is one of the more ancient families of flowering plants. Many palms are insect-pollinated, but a few are wind-pollinated. Date palms,[71,72] including the Canary Island date *(Phoenix canariensis)*, and queen palms *(Arecastrum romanzoffianum)*[70] are mildly allergenic and produce copious pollen locally. Their light yellow blooms can occur up to three times per year. The Everglades palm *(Acoelorrhaphe wrightii)* is also wind-pollinated.

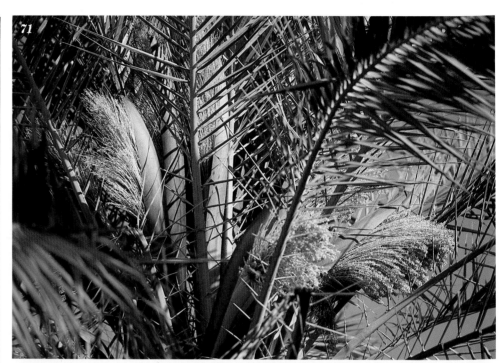

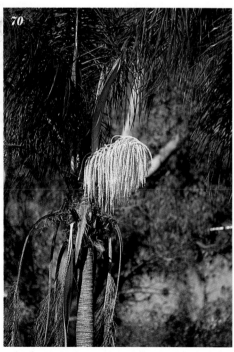

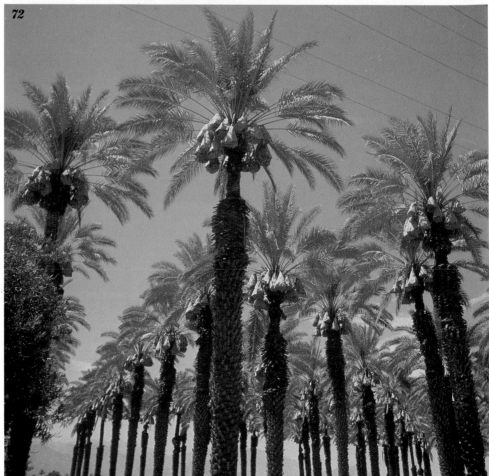

(70) Queen plam with straw-colored bloom. Note cement-like trunk of tree. **(71)** Wild date palm *(Phoenix sylvestris)* in bloom (male). **(72)** Date palm grove in California *(P. dactylifera)*.

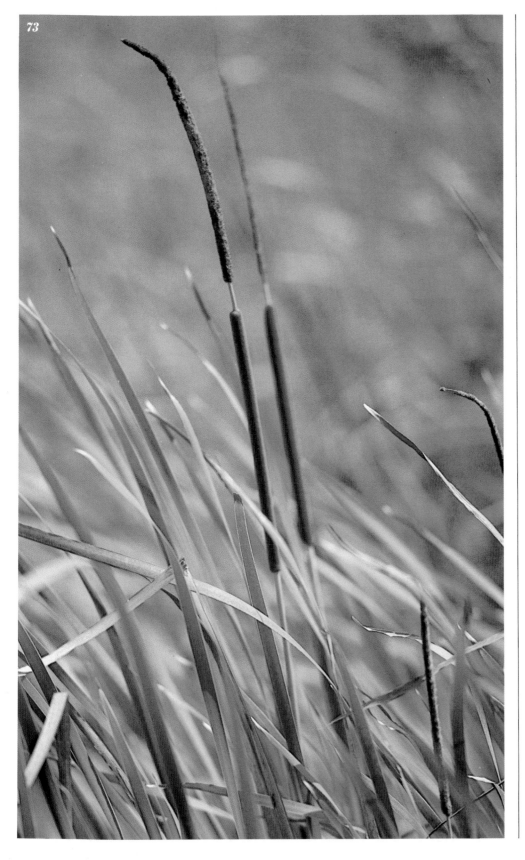

73

The Cattail Family

Cattails *(Typha)* are fresh-water marsh plants that grow up to ten feet tall. They have coarse, grasslike leaves and produce a single, pithy spike, with cylindrical, chocolate-brown flowers at the top 12 inches. The male bloom is located immediately above the fatter female bloom.[73] Cattails are common in all of the U.S., except at higher elevations. They bloom all summer. The pollen is airborne but is not a strong allergen. A home can become contaminated by a dry arrangement of cattails.

(73) Cattail with male bloom at top, female at bottom of spike.

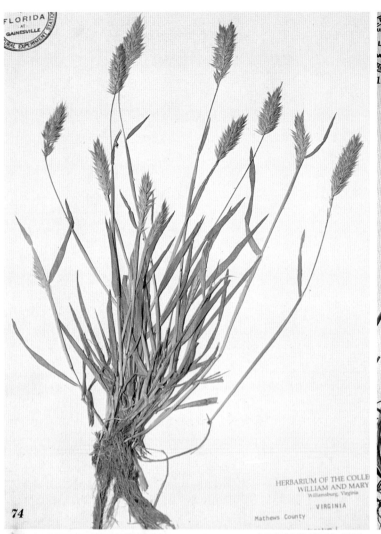

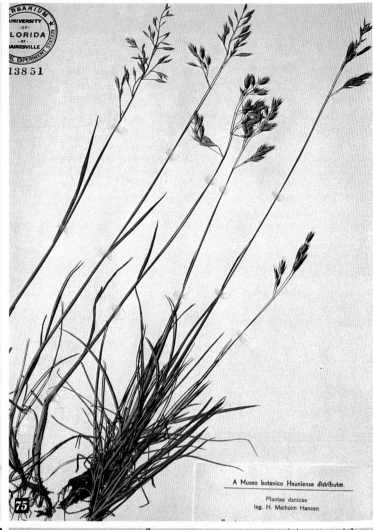

HERBARIUM OF THE COLLE
WILLIAM AND MARY
Williamsburg, Virginia

VIRGINIA

Mathews County

74

13851

A Museo botanico Hauniense distributæ.

Plantae danicae
leg. H. Mølholm Hansen

75

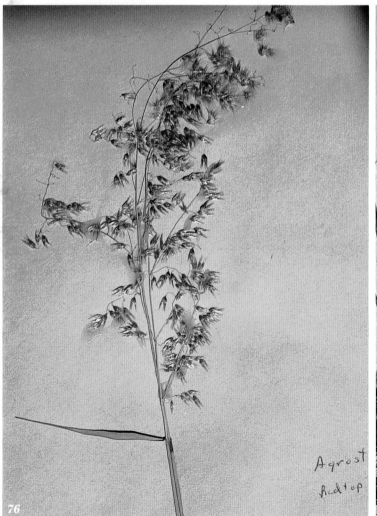

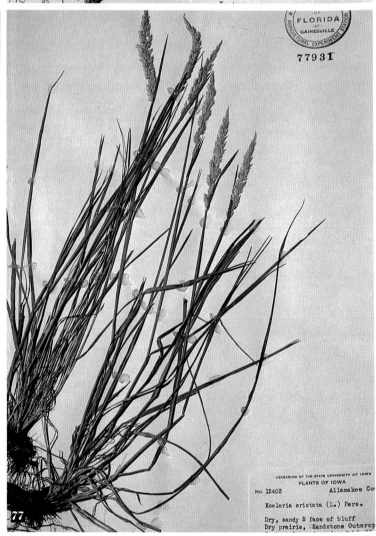

Agrost

Red top

76

77931

HERBARIUM OF THE STATE UNIVERSITY OF IOWA
PLANTS OF IOWA

No. 12403   Allamakee Cou

Koeleria cristata (L.) Pers.

Dry, sandy S face of bluff
Dry prairie, Sandstone Outcrop

77

32

Grasses

The most important allergenic plants in Europe are the grasses, which are members of the largest family of wind-pollinated plants. There are over 1200 species of grasses native to North America, but only a few of these are significant allergenic plants.

The bulk of airborne grass pollen in northern states is seen in June. Sweet vernal (*Anthoxanthum odo-ratum*),[74] a fragrant grass, is the earliest grass to bloom in the north. Its season is early May to mid-June. Orchard grass (*Dactylis glomerata*)[78] follows in those areas from late May to late June.

The blue or June grasses (*Poa*)[79] are widespread in the Midwest and plains states and the Northeast. They bloom in May and June, with Canada bluegrass (*Poa compressa*) blooming from June to August in Canada. Fescue (*Fes-*

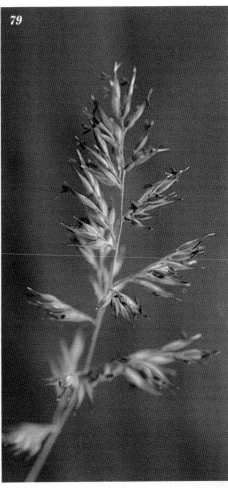

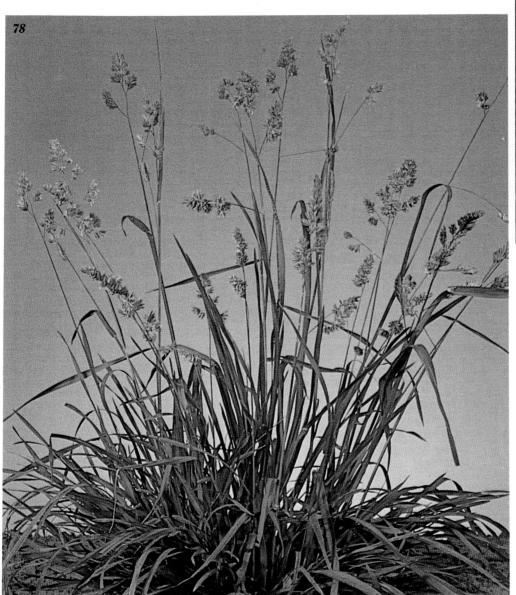

(74) Sweet vernal grass (dried specimen) is the first to bloom among the early northern grasses. It has a sweet fragrance. (75) Red fescue. (76) Redtop grass (*Agrostis stolonifera*). (77) Western June grass (*Koeleria*). (78) Orchard grass. (79) Bluegrass (*Poa pratense*).

Grasses *(continued)*

tuca),[75] timothy *(Phleum),*[80,81] and redtop *(Agrostis)*[76] bloom from June to July.

Perennial rye *(Lolium),*[82] the most important late grass on the Pacific Coast, blooms from July to August.

Earlier in the season in the Pacific area are sweet vernal, fescue, bluegrass, rye, velvet grass *(Holcus),* western June or hairgrass *(Koeleria)*[77] and timothy.[80,81]

In the southern states, Bermuda grass *(Cynodon)*[83,84] is nearly a year-round allergy threat. Johnson grass *(Sorghum)*[86,87,88] and salt-

(80) Timothy grass.

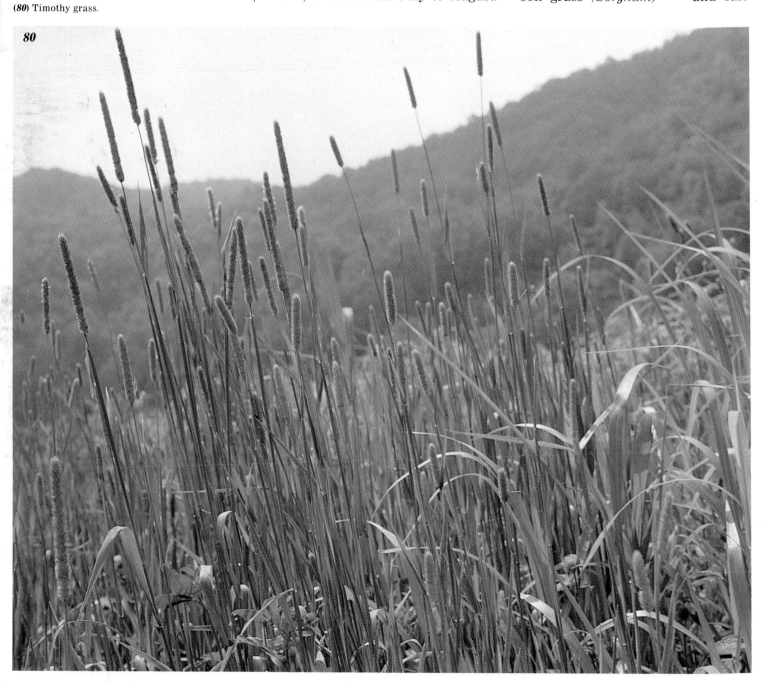

80

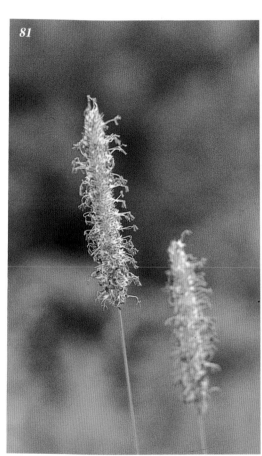

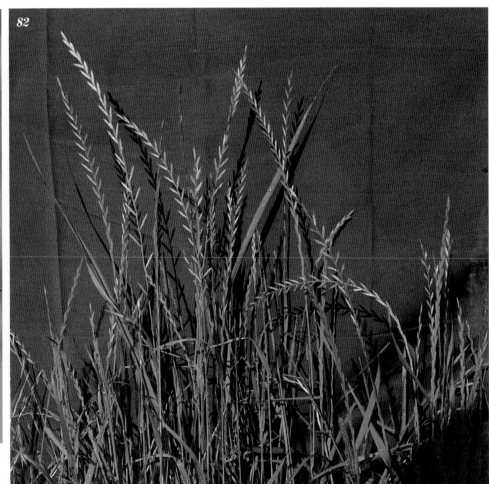

(81) Timothy grass, close-up of bloom. (82) Rye grass (*Lolium perenne*). (83) Bermuda grass (*Cynodon*). (84) Bermuda grass in harsh traffic.

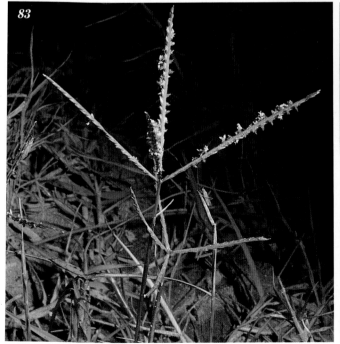

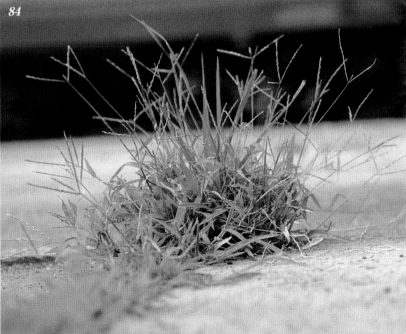

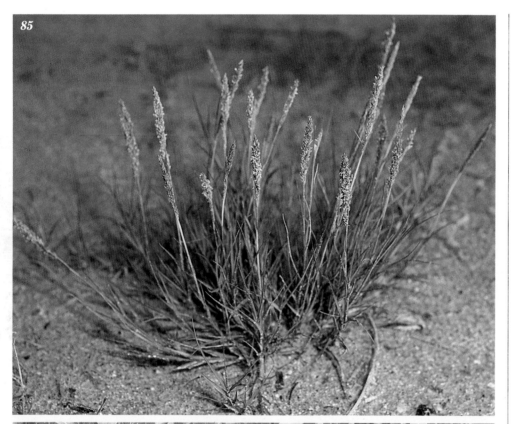

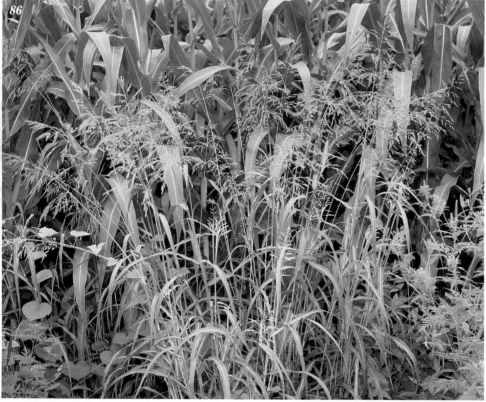

Grasses *(continued)*

grass *(Distichlis)*[85] also have long seasons in the South.

A simplified chart showing the pollen seasons for the most important allergenic grasses in different areas of the country is presented on page 62. However, there are many more grasses and the regions are more complex than presented.

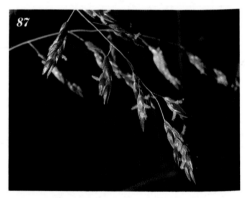

There may be as many as 20 active components in the pollen of a single species of grass. Rye, bluegrass, fescue, orchard grass, and timothy have very similar allergenic components. Brome, sweet vernal and bahia grasses are related to one another but not as closely as the rye group. Quack grass, saltgrass, and Bermuda grass are somewhat related, but they are more diverse in their allergenic components and only slightly resemble one another allergenically. Johnson, Sudan, and grama grasses are also a distinctive group. Sudan and Johnson grass are very closely related and yet have slight differences in their allergenic components.

The main active component of timothy grass has been found to cross-react with many other allergenic grasses, so some doctors only test for sensitivity to timothy,

(85) Saltgrass growing on beach.   **(86)** Johnson grass in front of cornfield.   **(87)** Johnson grass (close-up).

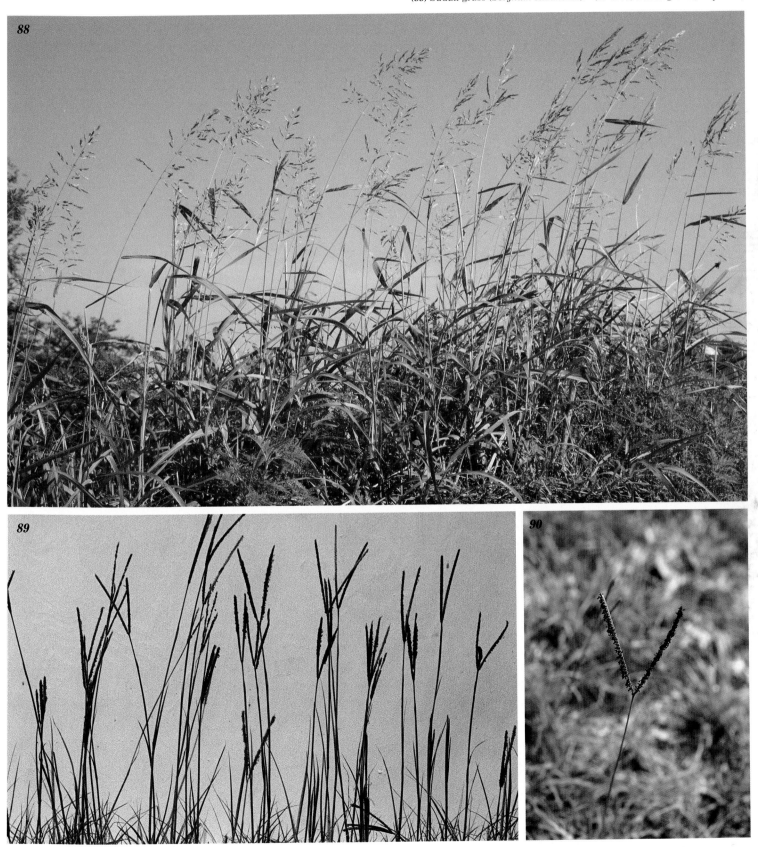

(88) Sudan grass (*Sorghum sudanense*). **(89 & 90)** Bahia grass (*Paspalum*).

37

Grasses *(continued)*

especially in the north. However, other grass allergens may be more potent for some individuals. A person who shows a reaction to timothy should still be tested for sensitivity to the other grasses of his area, especially Bermuda and bahia grasses, if he lives where these grasses are common.

Travel for business or pleasure can extend the period of time during which a person is exposed to grass allergens, because the grass to which the person is sensitive, or a related grass, may be blooming in the area visited at a different time than at home. Such prolonged exposure, even at low pollen counts, seems to cause more severe reactions than high counts for short periods.

Grass pollen in the air may incite a more severe allergic reaction by wheat-sensitive persons if they eat wheat at that time of the year.

The sedges[91] and rushes, two other grass-like groups, are almost all wind-pollinated. However, they are not considered to be important allergy provokers.

Very little of the pollen of St. Augustine grass *(Stenotaphrum secundatum)*[92] is airborne. However, the thick turf of this grass often harbors *Helminthosporium,* a mold that puts numerous allergenic spores into the atmosphere. The mold spores are thrown into the air when the grass is mowed.

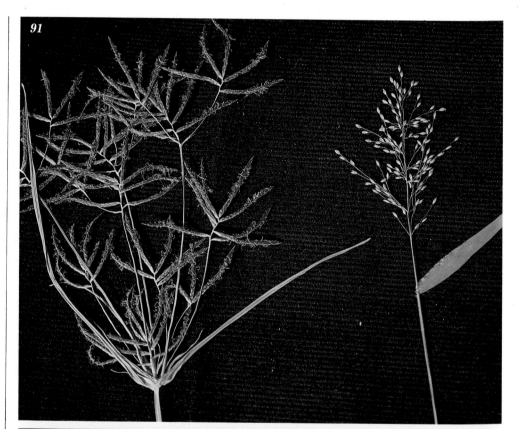

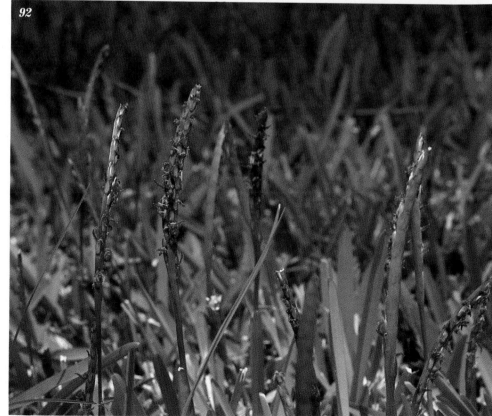

(**91**) A sedge (left) and panic grass (right), two non-allergenic plants. Sedges resemble grasses but belong to a different family. (**92**) St. Augustine grass. Its pollen does not become airborne, but this grass is a source of mold which grows on the leaves and stems. Mold spores are thrown into the air when the grass is mowed.

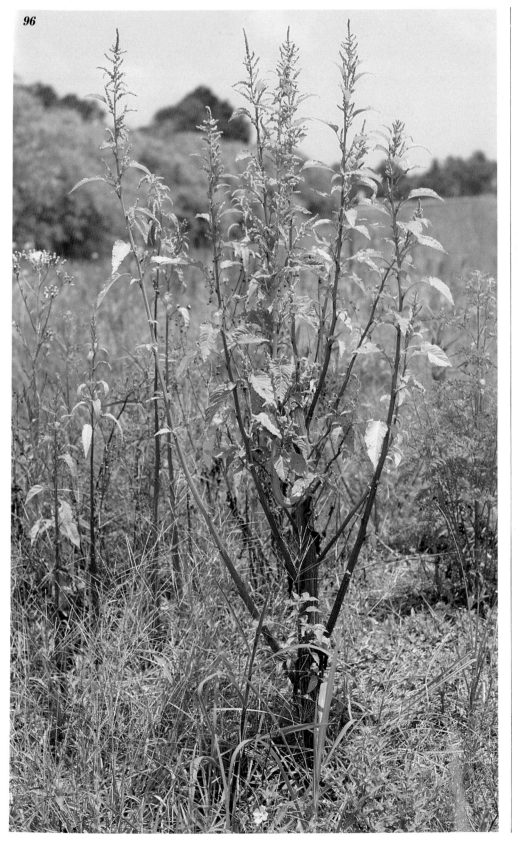

96

The Pigweed (Amaranthus) and Goosefoot (Chenopodium) Families

Pigweeds and goosefoots are typical weeds with rich, green, aggressive growth and inconspicuous flowers. They grow well in soils that are disturbed by farming or traffic. Their pollens are very similar in appearance, and the antigens of these plants cross-react so much that pollen surveys treat them as a single group. Some species are very large, such as the 28-foot southern water hemp (*Amaranthus australis*),[96] and some are small, such as the slender amaranth *(A. viridis)*.[97]

---

(96) Southern water hemp (*Amaranthus australis*). (97) Slender amaranth (*Amaranthus viridis*) growing from crack between asphalt and building in heavy traffic.

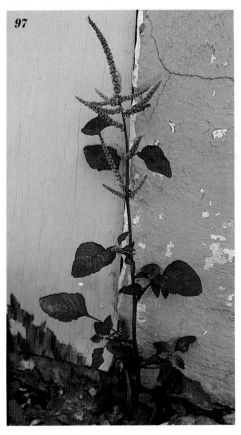

97

Dicots

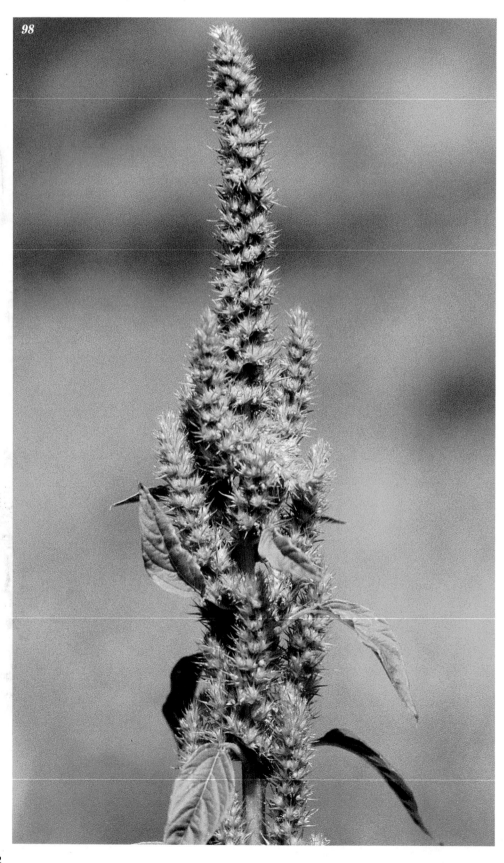

98

The Pigweed/Goosefoot Families *(continued)*

Other active allergenic species are redroot pigweed *(A. retroflexus),*[98] common pigweed *(A. hybridus),* Palmer's amaranth *(A. palmeri)* and western water hemp *(A. tamariscina).* They bloom from June to October, but may start in April in southern states.

The goosefoots are closely related to the pigweeds and bloom at the same times of year and in the same places. Lamb's quarter *(Chenopodium album)*[99] and Mexican tea *(C. ambrosioides)*[100] are very common throughout the U.S. Mexican tea is the most potent of these allergenic plants. Another very potent member is Russian thistle *(Salsola kali),*[101] which is not really a thistle. Russian thistle is from Eurasia and is the dominant tumbleweed[102] of dry waste places, especially in the western states. Its range is expanding eastward. It blooms from July to October.

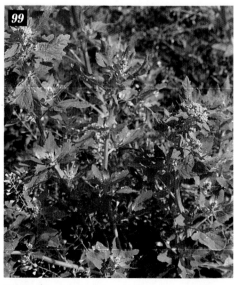

99

(98) Rough or redroot pigweed *(Amaranthus retroflexus).* **(99)** Lamb's quarter *(Chenopodium album).*

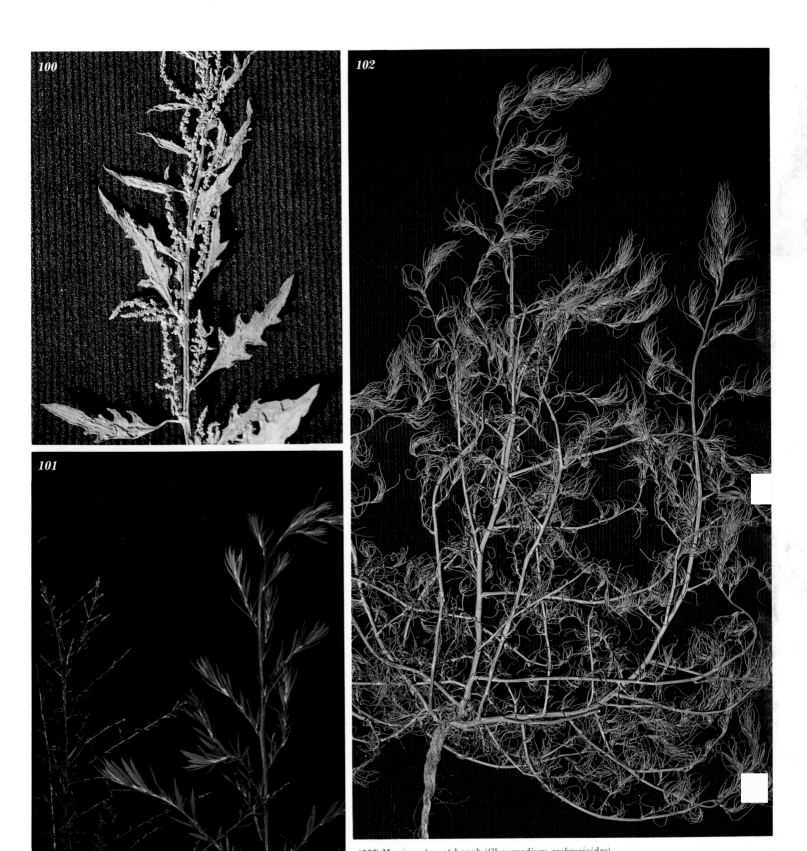

(**100**) Mexican tea at beach (*Chenopodium ambrosioides*).
(**101**) Branches of Russian thistle on left and burning bush on right.
(**102**) *Salsola kali* var. *tenuifolia*. Longer-leafed Russian thistle.

The Pigweed/Goosefoot Families *(continued)*

Kochia or burning bush *(Kochia scoparia)*[103,104] is another very potent allergenic weed which is common in the West. It is also found throughout the eastern states, contrary to the information in much of the literature. Burning bush blooms in dry places that are unsupportive of other plants.

Smother weed *(Bassia hyssopifolia)* and greasewood *(Sarcobatus vermiculatus)* are western weeds, and their pollens are significant allergens. Russian pigweed *(Axyris amaranthoides)*[105] and barilla *(Halogeton gomeratus)* are other members of the chenopods found among the western weeds.

The saltbushes, scales and orachs *(Atriplex)*[106,107] are found on dry, alkaline soils in the West. They

(103) Burning bush *(Kochia)* showing red color on stem which is the color of the plant in the fall.
(104) Disturbed land with burning bush.

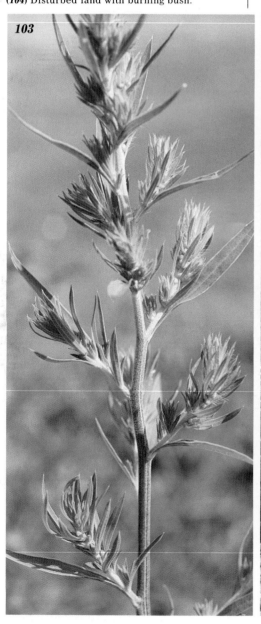

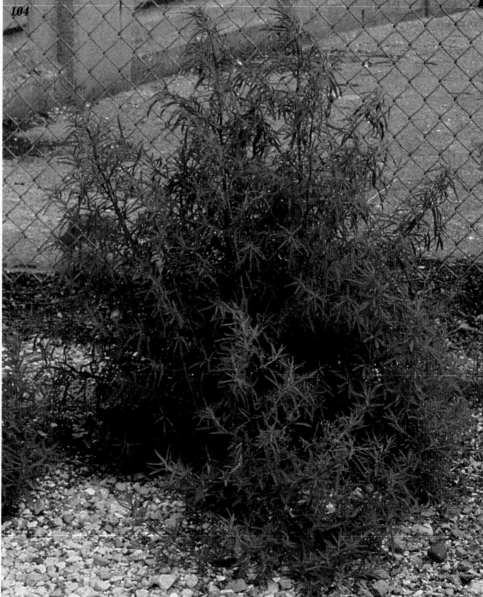

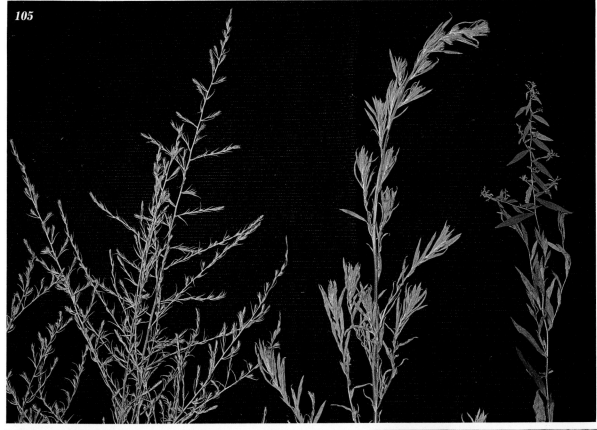

(105) Comparison of 3 related plants (left to right): Russian thistle (*Salsola kali*), burning bush (*Kochia scoparia*), and Russian pigweed (*Axyris*).
(106) Saltbush or sand atriplex (*Atriplex arenaria*). These plant parts are covered with tiny scales which help the plant survive the harsh conditions of the beach. **(107)** Blooms of sand atriplex, also known as seabeach orach.

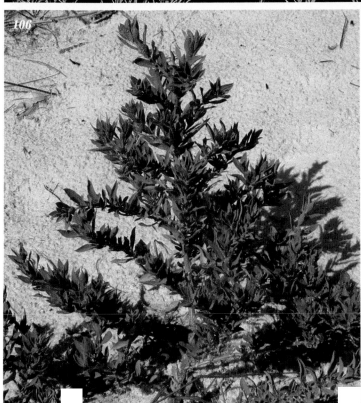

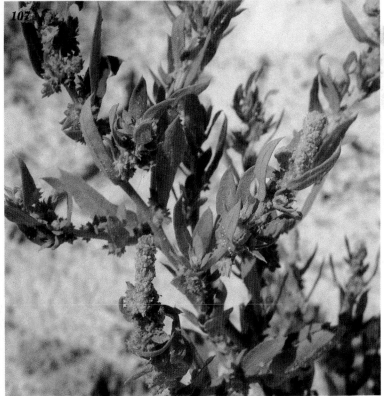

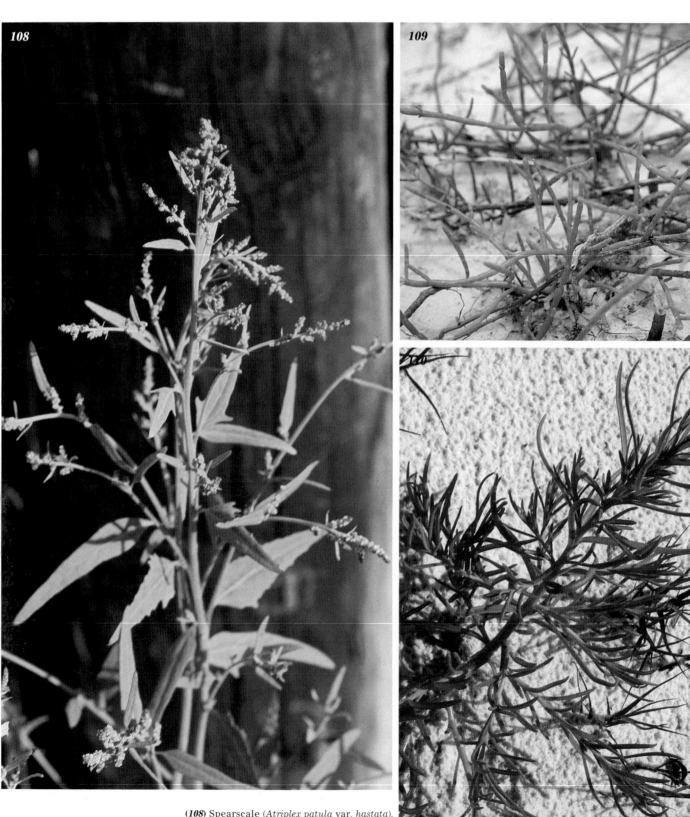

(**108**) Spearscale (*Atriplex patula* var. *hastata*).
(**109**) Glasswort (*Salicornia*) in bloom.
(**110**) *Suaeda linearis* (narrow-leafed sea blite) with
succulent leaves that conserve moisture.

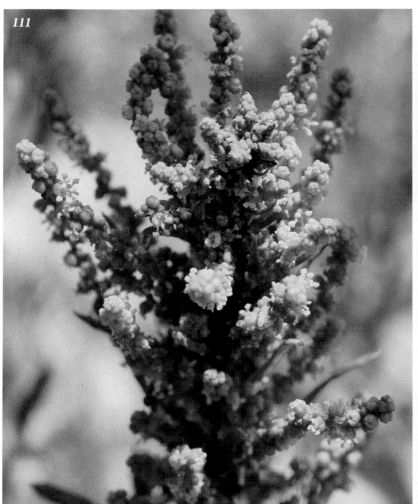

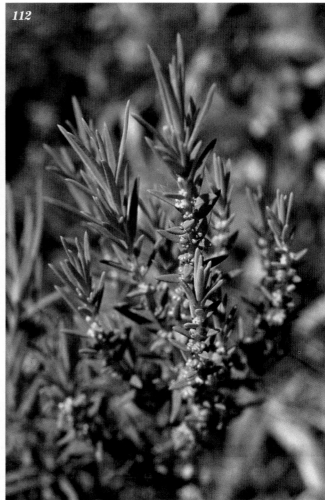

The Pigweed/Goosefoot Families (continued)

bloom in late summer and early fall, and their pollen cross-reacts with the pigweeds and goosefoots. Spearscale *(Atriplex patula)*[108] is a common coastal plant along with glasswort *(Salicornia)*,[109] sea blite *(Suaeda)*,[110,111] and saltwort *(Batis)*.[112]

Another plant whose pollen cross-reacts with the pigweed/goosefoot pollen is the sugar beet *(Beta vulgaris)*.[113] Sugar beets are grown commercially in Arizona, Utah and western Texas, blooming in May. The release of pollen has

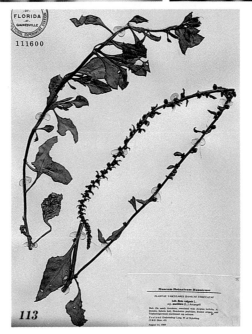

(111) Blooming *Suaeda maritima*. **(112)** Saltwort *(Batis maritima)* on beach. Saltwort is also used as the common name of *Salsola* (Russian thistle). **(113)** Sugar beet *(Beta vulgaris)* (a dried specimen folded to fit on a page). Note that the leaf and the bloom are both similar to pigweed. This plant is used for sugar and is prevalent in the Southwest.

been somewhat reduced since 1956 by the development and use of hybrids, but sugar beets still cause significant allergy problems in some areas.

Dicots

The Ragweed Family

The ragweed/composite family has been subdivided into 12-14 tribes:*

Heliantheae — sunflower
Ambrosieae — ragweed, cocklebur, marsh-elder, franseria
Helenieae — sneeze-weed, marigold, feverfew
Arctotideae — African daisy
Calenduleae — calendula
Inuleae — everlasting, straw flower
Astereae — aster, goldenrod, groundsel-bush, desert broom
Vernonieae — ironweed
Eupatorieae — dog fennel, joe-pye weed
Anthemideae — chamomile, yarrow, pyrethrum, chrysanthemum
Senecioneae — ragwort, butterweed
Cardueae — thistle, burdock
Mutisieae — gerbera daisy
Cichorieae — chicory, lettuce, dandelion

*The relationships and identification of the composites has been a great challenge to botanists and has caused more than one to shrug their shoulders and refer to them as "those darned yellow composites."

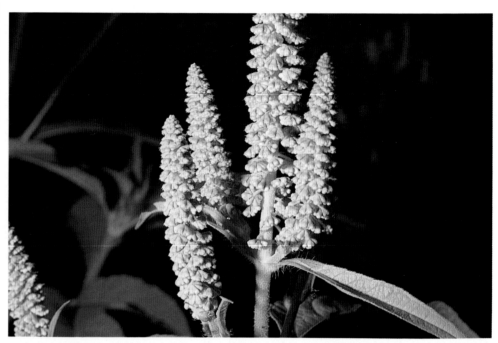

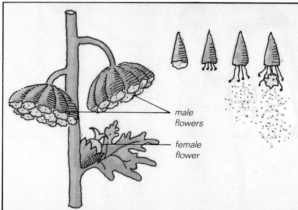

Lower Portion of Ragweed Spike.

The short, inconspicuous female flowers are few in number and are found where the upper leaves emerge from the stem. The male blooms consist of clusters of florets arranged like parasols along a spike. As the florets open, a piston sweeps the pollen from each one, ensuring that all the pollen will get blown away by the least little breeze. Few flowers are this efficient in dispersing pollen. One plant may produce one billion pollen grains.

male flowers

female flower

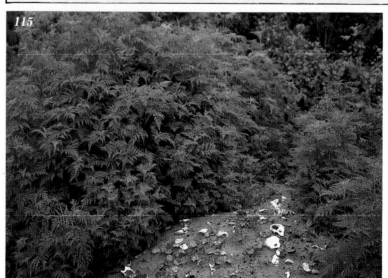

115

(114) Bloom of short ragweed (*Ambrosia artemisiifolia*) with male spike and small inconspicuous female flowers.
(115) Young short ragweed thriving in disturbed land near construction.

The scientific name of the ragweeds *(Ambrosia)* means "food of the gods." This name is an unlikely one for the most important allergenic plant of North America. It is a plant which is coarse, hairy, has a slightly noxious odor and no pretty flowers.

Prior to Colonial times, ragweeds were restricted to riverbanks, flood plains and naturally eroded areas. They grew far apart and survived by their great ability to produce large quantities of small, bouyant pollen.[114] As white men conquered and disturbed the land,[115] these plants became ever more dominant, especially in the Northeast and Midwest.

The giant ragweed *(Ambrosia trifida)*[116] stands a stately 12 feet tall. Short ragweed *(A. artemisiifolia)*[117] is found in all states, and it can bloom when only a few inches tall. Stressful growing conditions cause the plant to put its energy into its bloom, which it does by blooming profusely while skimping on foliage.[118] There are 17 species of ragweed in North America.

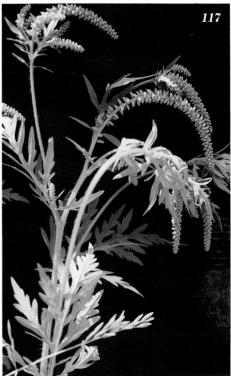

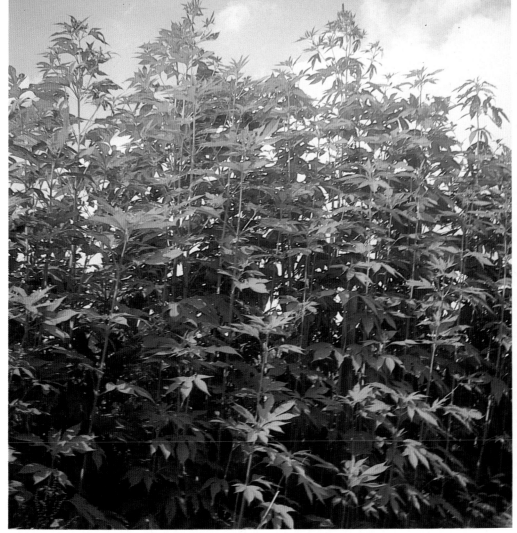

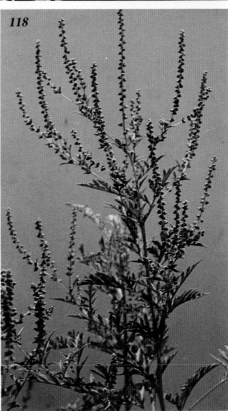

(*116*) Giant ragweed *(Ambrosia trifida)*. (*117*) Short ragweed. (*118*) Stressed ragweed blooming prolifically along highway.

49

The Ragweed Family *(continued)*

Ragweed starts blooming as days become shorter and nights longer, but pollen stops forming as night hours lengthen further and temperatures drop below 60 degrees F. Thus, in most areas ragweed blooms for about four to six weeks at nearly the same period each year (mid-July to September). The amount of pollen will increase with heavy spring rainfall and a hot dry pollen season, and it will decrease if spring does not provide good growing weather or if rain and humidity are too great during the blooming period. Giant ragweed does not release its pollen when humidity is over 70 percent.

There are multiple antigens in ragweed pollen, but the strongest, antigen E, is present in *Ambrosia* and *Franseria*.[119] The related sage-brushes *(Artemisia)* and marsh-elders *(Iva)* share some strong antigens with ragweed but do not have antigen E.

Burweed marsh-elder *(Iva xanthifolia)*[120] resembles giant ragweed except that its leaves are less cleft; it is present in the northeastern, midwestern and western states. Rough marsh-elder *(Iva ciliata)*[121] is similar in size but the spikes of the bloom are longer and have more bracts giving a coarser appearance. Rough marsh-elder is prevalent in the lower Mississippi Valley. Poverty weed *(Iva axillaris)* is only two feet tall, and grows in the western United States. Coastal marsh-elder *(Iva frutescens)*[122] and dune elder *(Iva imbricata)* are common in coastal areas. Marsh-elders are late summer and fall bloomers. Cocklebur *(Xanthium strumarium)* occasionally causes allergy problems, but its pollen is not abundant in the air.

Groundsel-bush *(Baccharis halimifolia)*[123,124] and desert broom *(Baccharis sarothroides)* are insect-pollinated, but a large amount of pollen gets into the air and causes allergy. The groundsel-bush is prevalent along the Atlantic and Gulf coasts from Massachusetts to Texas, and desert broom occurs in the western states. The female and male blooms are on separate plants.[124] Much wind pollination occurs as well as insect pollination.

(119) Bur ragweed *(Franseria discolor)*. Note burs (seeds with spines) and white-woolly fine hairs on leaves. This is a western weed.
(120) Burweed marsh-elder *(Iva xanthifolia)* Note that this plant stands stately like giant ragweed, but the larger leaves have no deep clefts, and are more like cocklebur leaves.

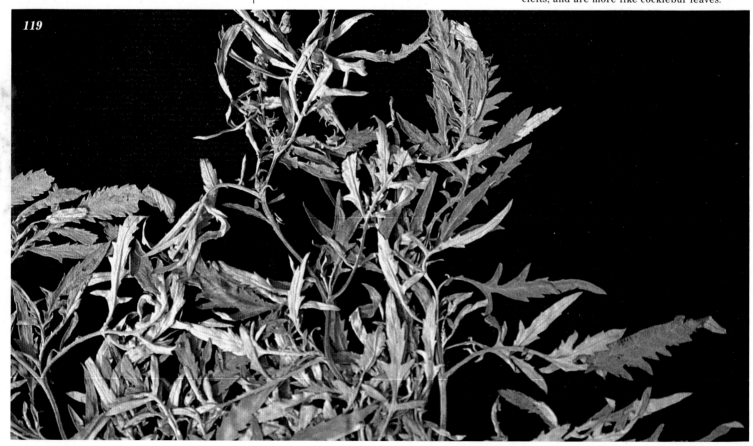

119

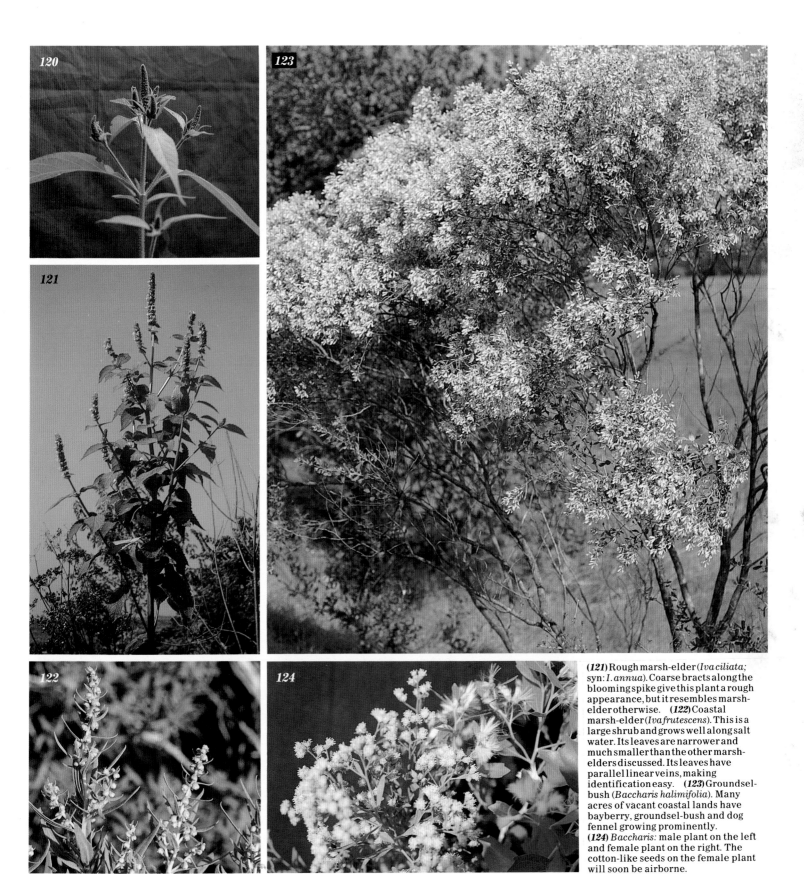

(121) Rough marsh-elder (*Iva ciliata*; syn: *I. annua*). Coarse bracts along the blooming spike give this plant a rough appearance, but it resembles marsh-elder otherwise.   (122) Coastal marsh-elder (*Iva frutescens*). This is a large shrub and grows well along salt water. Its leaves are narrower and much smaller than the other marsh-elders discussed. Its leaves have parallel linear veins, making identification easy.   (123) Groundsel-bush (*Baccharis halimifolia*). Many acres of vacant coastal lands have bayberry, groundsel-bush and dog fennel growing prominently.
(124) *Baccharis:* male plant on the left and female plant on the right. The cotton-like seeds on the female plant will soon be airborne.

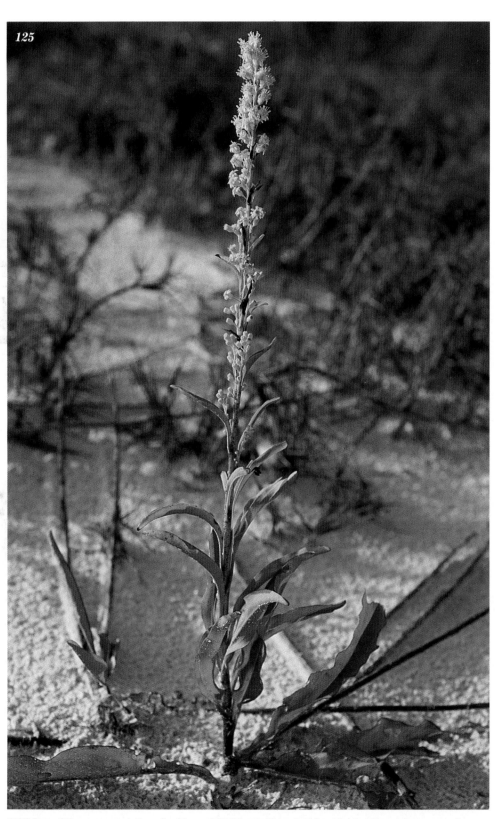

The Ragweed Family *(continued)*

The pound cake weed, or feverfew (*Parthenium hysterophorus*),[68][126] is an aggressive weed that has been found in the truck farming area near Homestead, Florida, since the 1970s. It is a cause of severe allergic contact skin reactions which were also noted in India and Australia. Another species, guayule *(P. argentatum)*, is being experimentally grown at EPCOT. This could possibly pose a serious health problem. Feverfew has been found to cause inhalant allergy problems for some people.

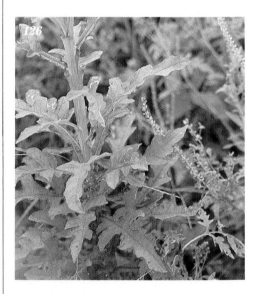

Many ragweed patients have blamed the conspicuous goldenrods *(Solidago)*[125] for allergies, but they are innocent, being insect-pollinated. The large, spiny pollen of goldenrod is seldom found in air surveys.

Dog fennel (*Eupatorium capillifolium*)[127,128] is partly insect-pollinated, but a great amount of pollen is also airborne. Baccharis and dog fennel bloom from late summer to December in the South, long after the ragweed season, and their pollen is almost

(125) One of the many varieties of goldenrod (*Solidago*). This plant is unfairly blamed for ragweed's effects because both plants bloom at about the same time. **(126)** Pound cake weed or feverfew (*Parthenium hysterophorus*) thrives in rainy climates and causes a skin reaction on contact.

indistinguishable from ragweed pollen.

Anthemis cotula[129] is also called dog fennel and is entirely insect-pollinated. It has daisy-like flowers and an unpleasant scent. Its extract will give a number of significant reactions, probably because it shares antigens with other composites, which are the real allergenic plants. Because of this sharing, some of the more colorful, insect-pollinated composites have given rise to serious allergic reactions. Eating sunflower seeds, drinking chamomile tea, and smelling pyrethrum insecticide, marigolds, or chysanthemums have all been reported to cause allergic reactions.

Even honey containing the pollens of these composites has caused suffering. It has been suggested that eating honey will "cure" allergy, but this is not recommended. The pollen in honey is not known, not very controllable, and has caused allergic reactions.

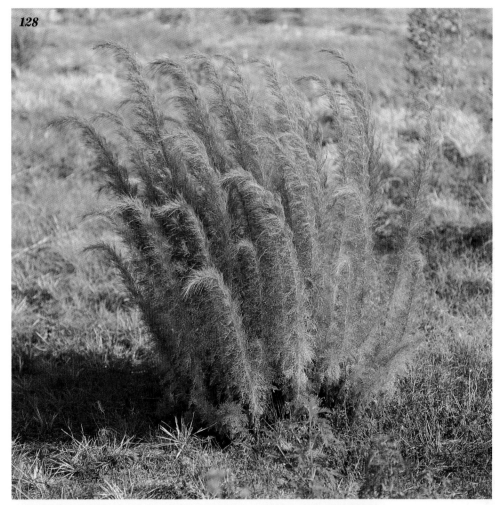

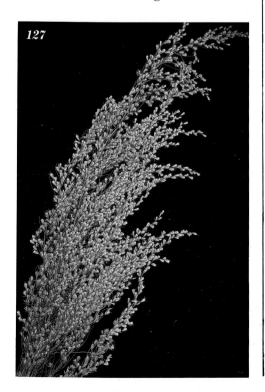

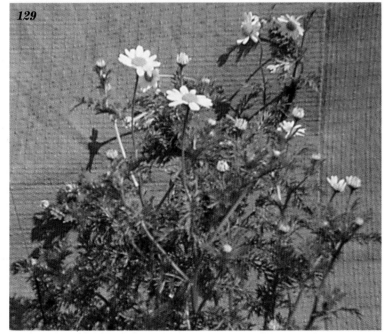

(127) Dog fennel bloom (close-up).
(128) Dog fennel (*Eupatorium capillifolium*). Note feathery appearance.
(129) *Anthemis cotula*, also called dog fennel.

The Ragweed Family *(continued)*

Sagebrush *(Artemisia tridentata)*[130] blooms from July to late September, and its pollen is a strong inhalant allergen of the western states. There are a number of other species of *Artemisia*[131] in the West and they all share similar antigens. The wormwoods *(A. biennis, A. annua, A. absinthium)*[132] and mugwort *(A. vulgaris)*[133] are prevalent in the central states, especially Tennessee, producing pollen in the late summer and fall.

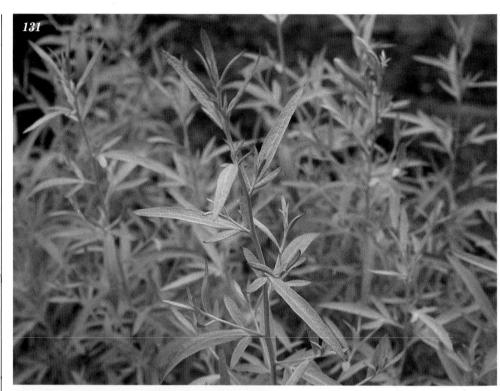

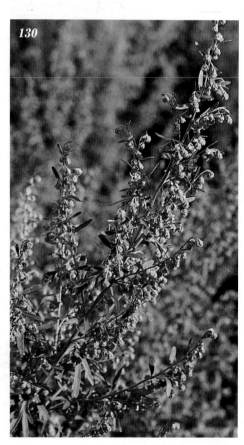

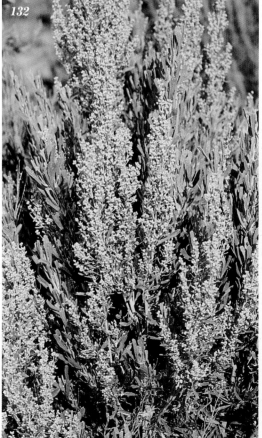

(130) Big sagebrush *(Artemisia tridentata)*. **(131)** Western mugwort *(Artemisia ludoviciana)*. A garden variety. **(132)** Wormwood *(Artemisia absinthium)*. **(133)** Mugwort *(Artemisia vulgaris)*. Note the fine, silvery-gray hairs on underside of leaf, a common finding in the sagebrush group. The leaf is deeply cleft, much like short ragweed, but the bloom is dumpy compared to the stately spike of ragweed.

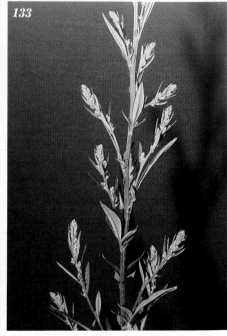

By being aware that the allergenic components of many composites are related to one another and may produce cross-reactions, a person may be able to avert serious illness. As mentioned earlier, contact dermatitis does occur with skin exposure to many composites.

The Hemp and Hop Family

Hemp or marijuana *(Cannabis)*[134] was planted in the Midwest during World War II for fiber to make rope. It has become common, even after attempts to rid the area of it because of its notoriety for drug abuse. The pollen is present from June to early October. Unfortunately, the smoke from the weed has more carcinogens than tobacco and is often contaminated with *Aspergillus* mold, which can cause a very serious lung disease. Hop *(Humulus)* is grown in the Northwest, and the pollen is similar to hemp and found in the air from July to August.

(134) Hemp *(Cannabis)* with female near post, the male more prominent on the right at border of corn field.

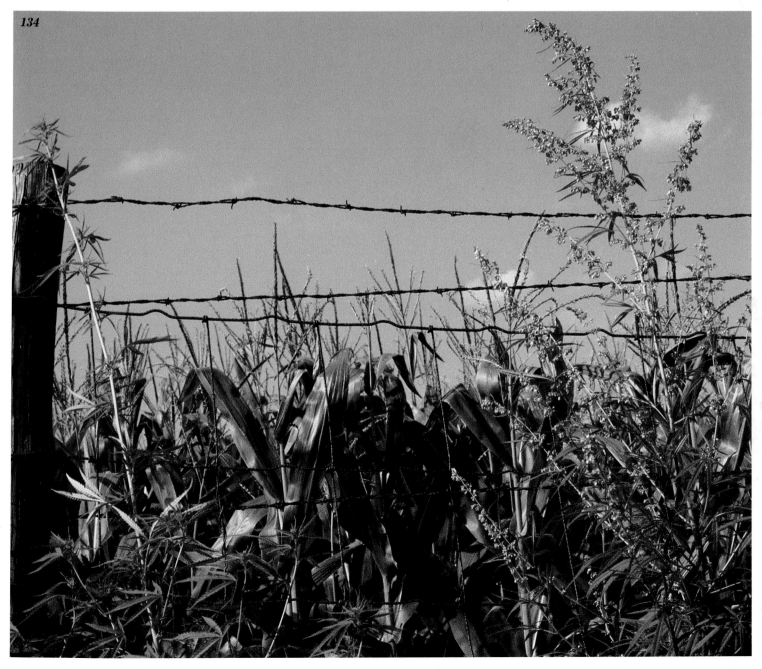

134

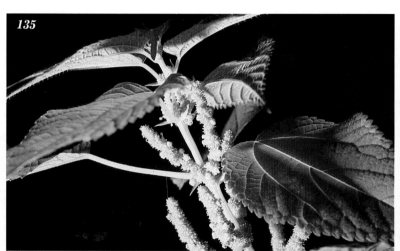

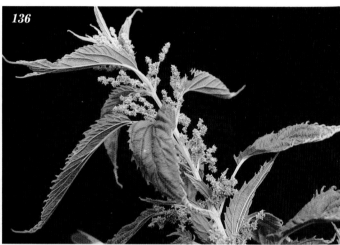

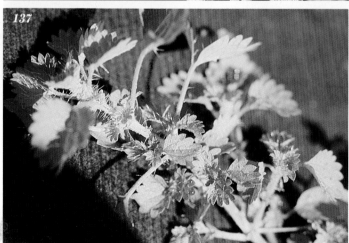

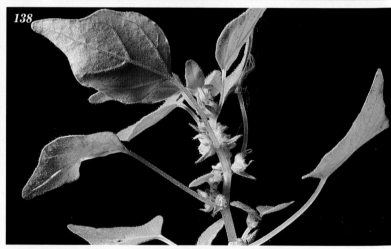

The Hemp and Hop Family
(continued)

Nettles[135,137] are loosely related to hemp and hop. The pollen is quite small. These smaller pollens were under-represented in past air surveys when gravity-slides were used. In Europe, nettles and pellitory[138,139] are important allergy plants. Nettle *(Urtica)* and pellitory *(Parietaria)* antigens do not cross-react. Pellitory is a shade-loving weed, like clearweed *(Pilea)*,[136] another member of the nettle family. Nettles, pellitory, and clearweed actively eject puffs of pollen into the air. They are present throughout the U.S.

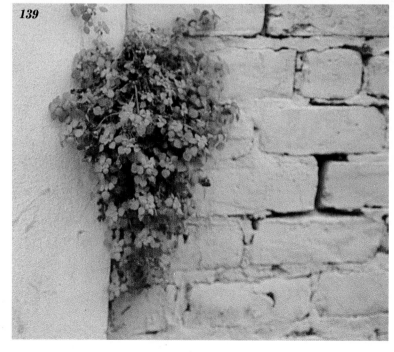

(135) False nettle *(Boehmeria)*, a common weed of the nettle family.
(136) Clearweed *(Pilea pumila)*. This member of the nettle family has no stinging hairs, but it is wind-pollinated.
(137) Wood nettle *(Laportea)* has active stinging hairs.
(138) Florida pellitory *(Parietaria floridana)* is prevalent in shady areas.
(139) Europeans call this plant "wall pellitory." This specimen was growing out of a crack in a wall in New Orleans. It can grow almost anywhere.

The Spurge Family

The spurge family has many diverse members, including the common weedy spurge[142] that creeps through bare areas of grass, crown-of-thorns, and poinsettias[140] or Christmas flowers. Most have milky sap that is irritating to the skin. The three-seeded mercury *(Acalypha rhomboidea)*[141] and the castor bean plant *(Ricinus communis)*[67] are the wind-pollinated members. They bloom in the summer. Dust from the processing of the oil and pomace of the caster bean is one of the most potent and dangerous allergens and causes castor bean dust allergy.

(140) Wild poinsettia. The white latex (sap) is irritating to the skin. *(141)* Three-seeded mercury *(Acalypha rhomboidea)*. Note that male and female blooms are separate but side by side; the male bloom is a longer spike-like shape. *(142)* Close-up of creeping spurge, a weed which often grows where grass cannot grow.

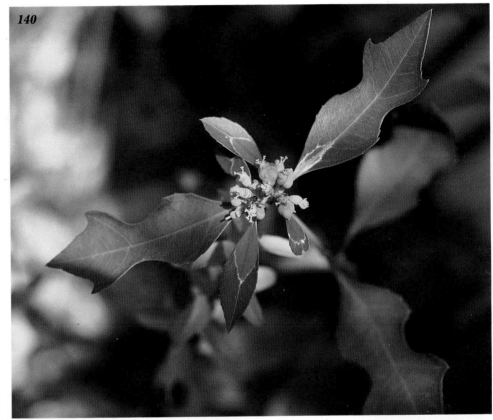

140

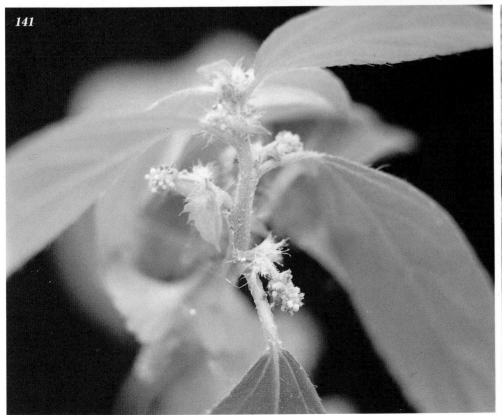

141

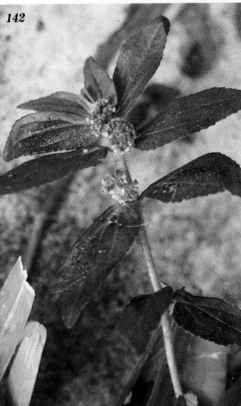

142

DUST ALLERGENS

House dust allergy is a most common problem in all areas except in dry, high altitudes. The dust mite, a microscopic organism, is the chief allergen in house dust. Upholstered furniture and rugs are common sources of dust mites, which are more prevalent in humid, warm climates. People allergic to dust mites should avoid rugs, upholstery, and feather pillows. In addition, the use of air conditioning to filter the air and dehumidify the home will decrease house dust mites. Mites feed upon dead skin cells, cereal grains, and molds; therefore, it is wise to keep the house free of these. Pets shedding skin cells promote more dust mites as well as the danders (skin cells) which cause animal allergies.

Chocolate and coffee bean dusts are also strong allergens and should be avoided by individuals with allergy histories. Cottonseed and flaxseed are very strong allergens and their dusts are associated with processing animal feeds, mattresses, upholstery, and the flour of cottonseed and flaxseed meals used for baking. Avoiding occupations associated with these materials will be helpful to many allergy-prone individuals.

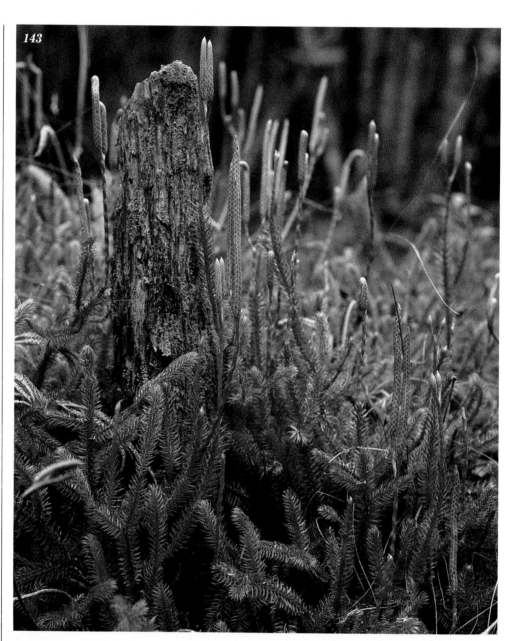

(143) Club moss (*Lycopodium*) of the piney woods has club-like spikes which give off spores.

SPORES

Club Moss (*Lycopodium*)

Club moss[143] is a tiny evergreen herb that grows in moist, shady woods and looks like a tiny pine tree only 5 to 10 inches tall. It has club-like cones that stand straight up like candles and shed large quantities of microscopic spores. These spores have been harvested for a powder for pharmaceuticals and theatrical make-up. They are highly flammable and are used in fireworks and stage productions for artificial lightning. Hikers are often exposed to the plants and their spores in late summer as they walk in cool woods in the Carolinas, Michigan, and the Pacific Northwest.

Ferns

Ferns[144] produce many spores, usually on the undersides of the leaves. These spores have a powdery brown or golden appearance, and they are abundant in air samples in summer and autumn. Some people are allergic to them.

(144) Fern leaves with sori (clusters of spore cases) on the undersides of the leaves. The larger leaf is a common polypody and the smaller is a sword fern.

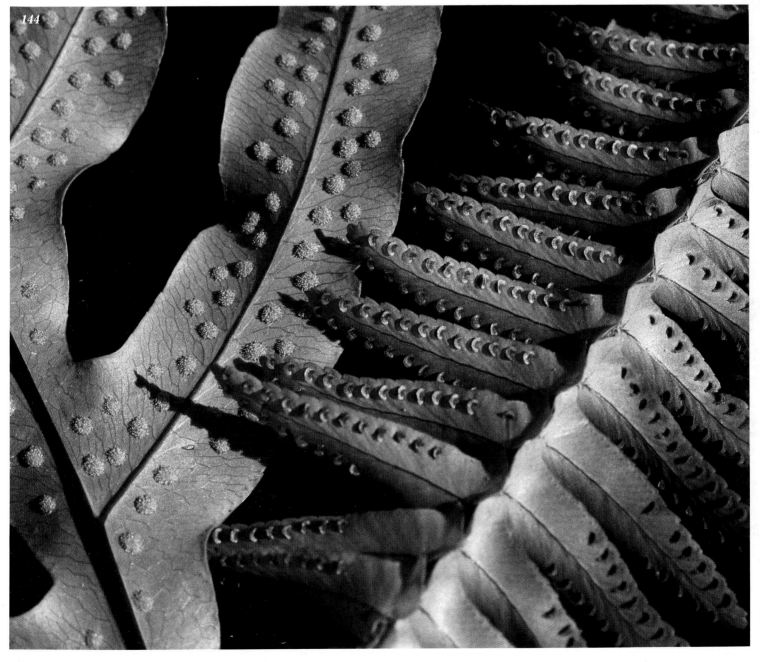

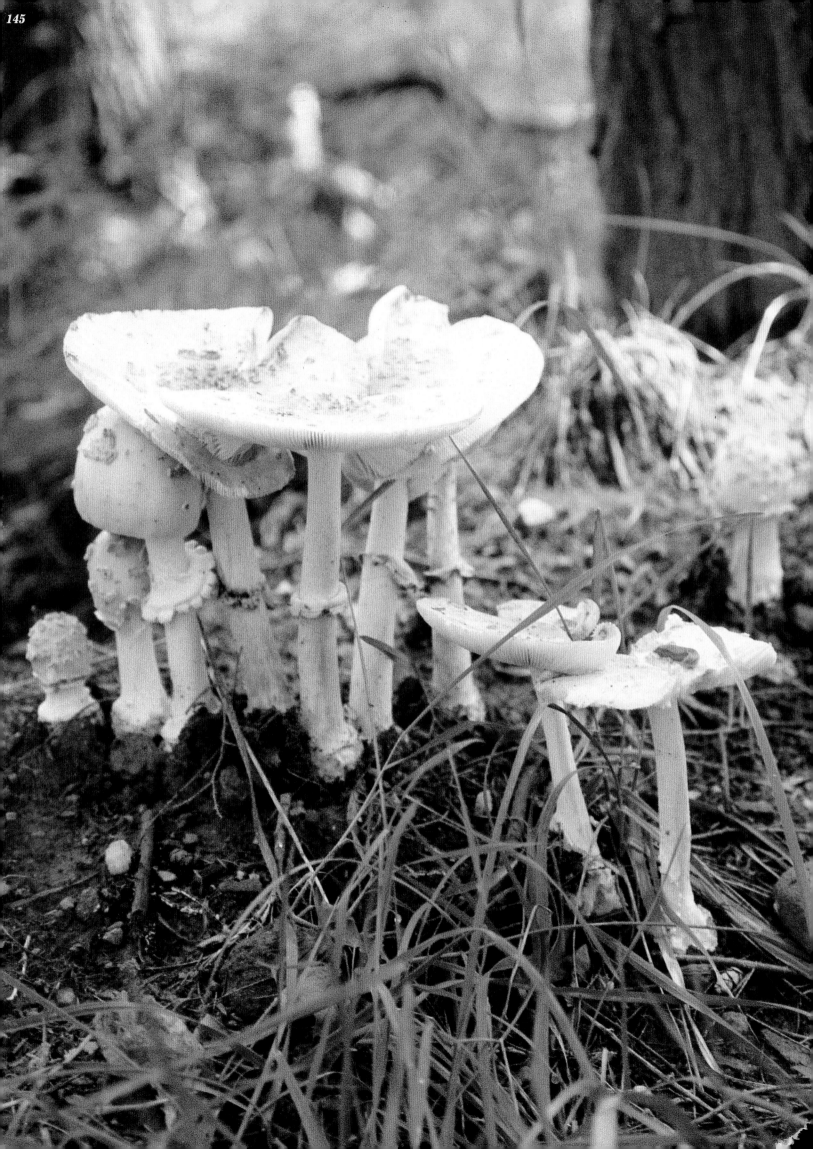

(145) Mushrooms: avoid kicking them and spreading the spores if you are allergic to molds. (146) Rotting orange with wild *Penicillium* mold.

Fungi

In many climates, for each pollen grain in the air there are 1000 mold spores. These are most numerous in the warmer months, and they are strong allergens. A mold[145] or a fungus is a plant without flowers or leaves that gets nourishment by feeding on organic matter. Mushrooms,[145] toadstools, rusts, smuts, molds, and yeasts are fungi. The term mold refers to those fungi with mycelial (filamentous or furry) growths. Fungi reproduce by spores which are one-celled, tough-walled structures, produced in very large numbers, that are able to survive in unfavorable conditions. Mold exposure increases with cutting the grass, raking dead leaves, or working with hay or mulch piles. Mushrooms have many spores under their "caps," and mold sensitive persons should avoid the temptation of kicking puffballs or toadstools.

DANDERS AND FEATHERS

Animal skin cells (danders) and feathers should be avoided within the home. Casual exposure outdoors often can be tolerated, but concentrating these materials in the home can lead to an unsolvable problem. The pet is easy to remove from the home, but his danders may be very difficult to remove after years of accumulation. Initially, the pet may be tolerated, but as time passes, a strong allergy may develop.

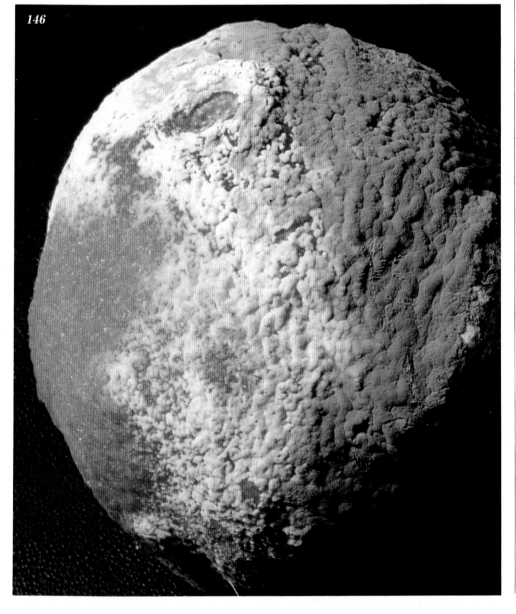

146

GRASS POLLEN SEASONS

	Jan	Feb	Mar	Apr	May	Jun	Jul	Aug	Sep	Oct	Nov	Dec
NORTHEAST												
sweet vernal					■	■	■					
orchard					■	■						
redtop						■	■	■	■			
bluegrass						■	■	■	■			
rye						■	■					
fescue						■	■					
timothy							■	■				
MIDWEST												
redtop					■	■	■	■	■			
brome					■	■	■	■	■			
orchard					■	■						
fescue					■	■	■					
bluegrass					■	■	■					
rye					■	■						
timothy						■	■					
grama							■	■				
sorghum							■	■	■			
NORTHWEST												
sweet vernal				■	■	■	■					
fescue					■	■	■					
bluegrass				■	■	■	■					
rye					■	■						
hairgrass					■	■	■					
redtop						■	■	■				
brome						■	■					
orchard						■	■					
velvet						■	■					
timothy						■	■					
SOUTHWEST												
Bermuda				■	■	■	■	■	■	■		
saltgrass					■	■	■					
grama						■	■	■				
brome					■	■	■					
fescue						■	■	■				
bluegrass						■	■					
sorghum						■	■	■	■			
SOUTHEAST												
Bermuda		■	■	■	■	■	■	■	■	■	■	■
saltgrass			■	■	■	■	■	■	■	■	■	■
bahia				■	■	■	■	■	■	■	■	■
redtop				■	■	■	■	■	■	■		■
fescue				■	■	■	■	■	■	■	■	■
sorghum				■	■	■	■	■	■	■	■	■

Although this chart begins with January, similar charts in the technical books and journals usually begin with March, because that is the beginning of the pollen season in most temperate areas.

How to avoid airborne allergens

1. Do not pick and sniff allergenic plants or their relatives.

2. Avoid areas where and when the plants are blooming.

3. Close the windows and use air conditioning to filter the air during the blooming season. The small models do very little filtering and the ion chargers have not been proven effective to relieve allergic disease. HEPA* filters should be used in the air conditioning.

   Also, the air conditioner should not create irritating ozone in significant amounts. Most electrical devices, such as electric motors, create ozone with their sparks, but they can be designed to diminish the problem. Some manufacturers advertise this feature.

4. When sick with a virus or exposed to air pollution, avoid all of the allergenic plants as a preventative measure, since that is when you are most likely to become sensitized to a new allergen.

5. Do not allow smoking in any closed area where you are confined for lengthy periods. Bronchitis and chronic ear problems are twice as prevalent in children exposed to smoking as in those who are not.

6. During your particular allergy season, do not ride with the car windows open because you will be exposed to large volumes of air containing pollen.

Many allergic individuals become sensitive to multiple allergens. Sometimes it will require the expertise of an allergist to determine which allergens are important. Skin tests and laboratory tests can give false positive and negative information. For this reason, establishing a correlation between the timing of the symptoms and the exposure to the blooming plants is crucial to a definitive diagnosis and proper treatment. A meticulous history of symptoms must be obtained. Any plans for injecton therapy should be delayed until that is properly done. You can help the allergist obtain a more accurate history if you keep a diary of symptoms for a full calendar year.

HEPA is an abbreviation for High Efficiency Particulate Air Filters. These filters have an effective cleaning rate of 98% of all particles down to 0.5 microns in size in one hour's time in most homes.

INDEX TO PLANTS AND OTHER ALLERGENS

Acacia 25
Acalypha 57
Acer 10
Acoelorrhaphe 30
African daisy 48
agave 28
agrimony 28, 29
Agrostis 34
alder 12
Alnus 12
aloe 28
Amaranthus 41
Ambrosia 48,49,50
American elm 14
Anacardium 28
angiosperms 10
animal danders 61
Anthemis 53
Anthoxanthum 33
antigen E 50
arborvitae 8
Arecastrum 30
Artemisia 50,54
Arizona cypress 5
ash 21
aspen 11
aster 28,48
Atriplex 44,45,46,47
Australian pine 20
Axyris 44,45
Baccharis 50,51
bahia grass 36,37,38,62
bald cypress 5,6,7
barilla 44
Bassia 44
Batis 47
bayberry 18,19
beech 16
beefwood 20
Bermuda grass 34,35,36,38,62
Bermuda juniper 5
Beta 47
Betula 12
birch 12
black oak 16
black willow 11
blackjack oak 17
bluegrass 33,34,36,62
Boehmeria 56
box elder 10
Brazilian pepper 28,29
brome grass 36,62
Broussonetia 15
buckwheat 39
bur ragweed 50
burdock 48
burning bush 43,44,45
burweed marsh-elder 50
buttercup 28
butterweed 48
cajeput 27
Calendula 48

California scrub oak 17
Canary Island date palm 30
Cannabis 55
Carpinus 12
Carya 22
cashew 28
castor bean 28,29,57
Casuarina 20
catkin 11
cattail 31
cedar 4,5
cedar elm 14
cedar of Lebanon 4
celery 28
Celtis 14
chamomile 48
Chenopodium 41,42,43
chestnut 16
chestnut oak 17
chicory 48
chocolate 58
chrysanthemum 28,48,53
citrus 27,28
clearweed 56
club moss 58
Cnidoscolus 28
coast live oak 16
coast redwood 7,8
coastal marsh-elder 50,51
cocklebur 48
coffee bean 58
composite 28,48
Comptonia 19
conifers 4
Corchorus 26
Corylus 12
cottonseed 58
cottonwood 11
crown-of-thorns 57
curly dock 39
Cryptomeria 8
Cynodon 34,35
cypress 5,6,7
Dactylis 33
dandelion 48
dander 58,61
date palm 30
deodar cedar 4
desert broom 48,50
dicotyledons 10,39
Distichlis 36
dock 39
dog fennel 28,48,51,52,53
dune elder 50
dust mites 58
elm 14
English plantain 40
eucalyptus 27
Eupatorium 48,52
Euphorbia 28
Everglades palm 30
everlasting 48

false nettle 56
feathers 58,61
fern 59
fescue 33,34,36,62
Festuca 34
feverfew 28,29,48,52
fir 4
flaxseed 58
fleawort 40
Franseria 48,50
Fraxinus 21
fungi 61
gerbera daisy 48
giant ragweed 49
Ginkgo 9
glasswort 46,47
goldenrod 48,52
goosefoot 41,42,43,44,45,47
grama grass 36,62
grass 30,32-38,62
grass pollen seasons 62
greasewood 44
groundsel-bush 48,50,51
guayule 52
gymnosperms 4
hackberry 14
hairgrass 33,34,62
Halogeton 44
Hamamelis 24
hazel 12
hedge 15
Helminthosporium 38
hemlock 4
hemp 55
hickory 22
Holcus 34
honey 53
hop 55
hophornbeam 13
hornbeam 12
horse nettle 28
house dust mite 58
Humulus 55
ironweed 48
Iva 50,51
Japanese cedar 8
joe-pye weed 48
Johnson grass 36
Juglans 22
June grass 33,34
juniper 5
jute 26
Kochia 43,44,45
Koeleria 33,34
lamb's quarter 42
Laportea 56
larch 4,8
laurel oak 17
legume 25
lettuce 48
Ligustrum 21
linden 26

Liquidambar 24
live oak 16
Lolium 34,35
Lycopodium 58
Maclura 15
maidenhair tree 9
manchineel 28
Mangifera 28
mango 28
maple 10
marigold 28,48,53
marijuana 55
marsh-elder 28,48,50,51
Melaleuca 27
mesquite 25
Metopium 28
Mexican cedar 5
Mexican tea 42,43
mold spores 61
monocotyledons 30
Monterey cypress 5
Morus 15
mountain ash 21
mountain cedar 5
mugwort 54
mulberry 15
mushrooms 60,61
Myrica 19
myrtle oak 16
nettle 28,56
oak 16,17
oleoresin 28
olive 21
orach 44
orchard grass 33,36,62
osage orange 15
Ostrya 12
overcup oak 17
palm 30
Palmer's amaranth 42
panic grass 38
paper mulberry 15
Parietaria 56
Parthenium 29,52
Paspalum 36,37
pecan 22
pellitory 56
Penicillium 61
Phleum 34
Phoenix 30
pigweed 41,42,44,45,47
Pilea 56
Pinchot juniper 5
pine 4
Pinus 4
pistachio 28
Pistacia 28
planetree 23
Plantago 40
plantain 40
Platanus 23
Platycladus 8